Lotus Publishing
Chichester, England

North Atlantic Books
Berkeley, California

First published in 2007 by
Lotus Publishing
3. Chapel Street, Chichester, PO19 1BU and
North Atlantic Books
P O Box 12327
Berkeley, California 94712

Illustrations Amanda Williams
Line Drawings Chris Fulcher and Wendy Craig
Text Design Wendy Craig
Cover Design Jim Wilkie
Printed and Bound in the UK by Scotprint

The Anatomy of Sports Injuries is sponsored by the Society for the Study of Native Arts and Sciences, a nonprofit educational corporation whose goals are to develop an educational and cross-cultural perspective linking various scientific, social, and artistic fields; to nurture a holistic view of arts, sciences, humanities, and healing; and to publish and distribute literature on the relationship of mind, body, and nature.

British Library Cataloguing in Publication Data
A CIP record for this book is available from the British Library
ISBN 978 1 905367 06 1 (Lotus Publishing)
ISBN 978 1 55643 666 6 (North Atlantic Books)

Library of Congress Cataloguing-in-Publication Data
Walker, Brad, 1971-
  The anatomy of sports injuries / Brad Walker.
     p. ; cm.
  Includes bibliographical references and index.
  ISBN 978-1-55643-666-6 (North Atlantic Books : pbk.)
  1. Sports injuries--Atlases. I. Title.
  [DNLM: 1. Athletic Injuries--Atlases. 2. Athletic Injuries--Handbooks.
3. Athletic Injuries--therapy--Atlases. 4. Athletic
Injuries--therapy--Handbooks. QT 29 W177a 2007]
RD97.W35 2007
617.1'027--dc22
                        2007010564

Contents

Introduction   5

Chapter 1: Explanation of Sports Injury   7
What Constitutes a Sports Injury?   8
What is Affected in a Sports Injury?   8
Is the Sports Injury Acute or Chronic?   11
How Are Sports Injuries Classified?   11
How Are Sprain and Strain Injuries Classified?   12

Chapter 2: Sports Injury Prevention   13
Warm-up   14
Cool-down   17
The FITT Principle   19
Overtraining   20
Fitness and Skill Development   22
Stretching and Flexibility   33
Facilities, Rules, and Protective Devices   42

Chapter 3: Sports Injury Treatment
and Rehabilitation   43
Introduction to Sports Injury Management   44
Regaining the Fitness Components   48

Chapter 4: Sports Injuries of the Skin   53
001:   Cuts, Abrasions, Chafing   55
002:   Sunburn   56
003:   Frostbite   57
004:   Athlete's Foot (Tinea Pedis)   59
005:   Blisters   60
006:   Corns, Calluses, Plantar Warts (Verrucae)   61

Chapter 5: Sports Injuries of the
Head and Neck   63
Acute
007:   Head Concussion, Contusion,
          Haemorrhage, Fracture   65
008:   Neck Strain, Fracture, Contusion   67
009:   Cervical Nerve Stretch Syndrome   68
010:   Whiplash (Neck Sprain)   69
011:   Wryneck (Acute Torticollis)   71
012:   Slipped Disc (Acute Cervical
          Disc Disease)   73
013:   Pinched Nerve (Cervical Radiculitis)   74
014:   Spur Formation (Cervical Spondylosis)   75
015:   Teeth   77
016:   Eye   78
017:   Ear   79
018:   Nose   80

Chapter 6: Sports Injuries of the
Hands and Fingers   81
Acute
019:   Metacarpal Fractures   83
020:   Thumb Sprain (Ulnar Collateral Ligament)   84
021:   Mallet Finger (Long Extensor Tendon)   85
022:   Finger Sprain   87
023:   Finger Dislocation   88
Chronic
024:   Hand / Finger Tendinitis   89

Chapter 7: Sports Injuries of the
Wrists and Forearm   91
Acute
025:   Wrist and Forearm Fracture   93
026:   Wrist Sprain   94
027:   Wrist Dislocation   95
Chronic
028:   Carpal Tunnel Syndrome   97
029:   Ulnar Tunnel Syndrome   98
030:   Wrist Ganglion Cyst   100
031:   Wrist Tendinitis   101

Chapter 8: Sports Injuries of the Elbow   103
Acute
032:   Elbow Fracture   105
033:   Elbow Sprain   106
034:   Elbow Dislocation   107
035:   Triceps Brachii Tendon Rupture   109
Chronic
036:   Tennis Elbow   110
037:   Golfer's Elbow   111
038:   Thrower's Elbow   113
039:   Elbow Bursitis   114

Chapter 9: Sports Injuries of the
Shoulder and Upper Arm   115
Acute
040:   Fracture (Collar Bone, Humerus)   117
041:   Dislocation of the Shoulder   119
042:   Shoulder Subluxation   121
043:   Acromioclavicular Separation   122
044:   Sternoclavicular Separation   123
045:   Biceps Brachii Tendon Rupture   125
046:   Biceps Brachii Bruise   126
047:   Muscle Strain (Biceps Brachii, Chest)   127
Chronic
048:   Impingement Syndrome   129
049:   Rotator Cuff Tendinitis   130
050:   Shoulder Bursitis   131
051:   Bicipital Tendinitis   133
052:   Pectoral Muscle Insertion Inflammation   134
053:   Frozen Shoulder (Adhesive Capsulitis)   135

Chapter 10: Sports Injuries of the Back and Spine   137
Acute
054: Muscle Strain of the Back   139
055: Ligament Sprain of the Back   140
056: Thoracic Contusion   141
Chronic
057: Slipped Disc (Herniated or Ruptured)   143
058: Bulging Disc   144
059: Stress Fracture of the Vertebra   145

Chapter 11: Sports Injuries of the Chest and Abdomen   147
Acute
060: Broken (Fractured) Ribs   149
061: Flail Chest   151
062: Abdominal Muscle Strain   154

Chapter 12: Sports Injuries of the Hips, Pelvis, and Groin   155
Acute
063: Hip Flexor Strain   157
064: Hip Pointer   158
065: Avulsion Fracture   159
066: Groin Strain   160
Chronic
067: Osteitis Pubis   162
068: Stress Fracture   163
069: Piriformis Syndrome   165
070: Iliopsoas Tendinitis   167
071: Tendinitis of the Adductor Muscles   168
072: Snapping Hip Syndrome   169
073: Trochanteric Bursitis   171

Chapter 13: Sports Injuries of the Hamstrings and Quadriceps   173
Acute
074: Femur Fracture   175
075: Quadriceps Strain   177
076: Hamstring Strain   178
077: Thigh Bruise (Contusion)   179
Chronic
078: Iliotibial Band Syndrome   181
079: Quadriceps Tendinitis   183

Chapter 14: Sports Injuries of the Knee   185
Acute
080: Medial Collateral Ligament Sprain   187
081: Anterior Cruciate Ligament Sprain   188
082: Meniscus Tear   189
Chronic
083: Bursitis   191
084: Knee Synovial Plica   192
085: Osgood-Schlatter Syndrome   193
086: Osteochondritis Dissecans   195
087: Patellofemoral Pain Syndrome   196
088: Patellar Tendinitis (Jumper's Knee)   197
089: Chondromalacia Patellae (Runner's Knee)   199
090: Subluxing Knee Cap   200

Chapter 15: Sports Injuries of the Lower Leg   201
Acute
091: Fractures (Tibia, Fibula)   203
092: Calf Strain   205
093: Achilles Tendon Strain   206
Chronic
094: Achilles Tendinitis   207
095: Medial Tibial Pain Syndrome (Shin Splints)   209
096: Stress Fracture   210
097: Anterior Compartment Syndrome   211

Chapter 16: Sports Injuries of the Ankle   213
Acute
098: Ankle Sprain   215
099: Ankle Fracture   216
Chronic
100: Posterior Tibial Tendinitis   217
101: Peroneal Tendon Subluxation   219
102: Peroneal Tendinitis   220
103: Osteochondritis Dissecans   222
104: Supination   223
105: Pronation   224

Chapter 17: Sports Injuries of the Foot   225
Acute
106: Fracture of the Foot   227
Chronic
107: Retrocalcaneal Bursitis   228
108: Stress Fracture   229
109: Flexor and Extensor Tendinitis   231
110: Morton's Neuroma   233
111: Sesamoiditis   234
112: Bunions   236
113: Hammer Toe   237
114: Turf Toe   238
115: Claw Foot (Pes Cavus)   240
116: Plantar Fasciitis   241
117: Heel Spur   242
118: Black Nail (Subungual Haematoma)   243
119: Ingrown Toenail   244

Glossary of Terms   245
Resources   252
Index   253

Introduction

As sports participation rates increase, so does the occurrence of sport-related injury. As a consequence, there is a need for detailed, easy-to-understand references on the prevention, treatment, and management of sports injury.

Whilst there are many books that deal with this subject, very few are able to present detailed anatomical information in a way that is easy to understand for everyone from the weekend warrior to the professional athlete; from the first year personal trainer to the seasoned sports coach; or from the recent university graduate to the accomplished sports doctor.

This is where *The Anatomy of Sports Injuries* excels. By using a combination of real-life practical experience and theoretical book knowledge, the author is able to present complex prevention, treatment, and management strategies in a way that everyone can understand. The detailed, yet simple information will help the reader prevent sports injury from occurring, and in the event that an injury does occur, help to treat it effectively, to allow a return to activity in as little time as possible.

That's not all: *The Anatomy of Sports Injuries* goes one step further. By using full colour illustrations, the book is able to take the reader inside the body, providing a visual aid, which allows a greater understanding of the workings of the human body during the sports injury management process.

The Anatomy of Sports Injuries looks at sport-related injury from every angle. In Chapter 1, a general outline of what sports injury is and a number of definitions are provided. In Chapter 2, key prevention strategies are explained to help reduce the occurrence of sport-related injury. In Chapter 3, a comprehensive treatment and rehabilitation process is outlined to ensure a quick and complete recovery.

Finally, in Chapters 4–17, the ultimate strength of the book, a detailed overview of 119 sports injuries is provided in an easy-to-locate format. Divided into key areas of the body, each sports injury review outlines: the anatomy and physiology involved, possible causes, signs and symptoms, complications, immediate treatment, rehabilitation procedures, and long-term prognosis.

Aimed at fitness enthusiasts and health care professionals of any level, *The Anatomy of Sports Injuries* also provides suggested strength and flexibility exercises to aid with sports injury prevention, treatment, and rehabilitation. These exercises are by no means exhaustive, but merely provide guidance. Consult your health care professional for a tailor-made program to suit your own individual needs.

Note
There appears to be some confusion whether to refer to the patellar tendon, or the patellar ligament. The patellar ligament (ligamentum patellae) extends from the patella down to the tibial tuberosity. If one thinks of the patella as a bone in its own right, then it should naturally be called the patellar ligament, since it connects two bones (the patella to the tibia). However, if you consider the patella to be a sesamoid bone living within the quadriceps tendon, then calling it the patellar tendon also seems correct (connecting muscle to bone). Another suggestion might be that as a tendon ages, it becomes more ligamentous. So for clarity, I have referred to it as the patellar (tendon) ligament throughout.

Chapter

1

Explanation of Sports Injury

What Constitutes a Sports Injury?

What is Affected in a Sports Injury?

Is the Sports Injury Acute or Chronic?

How Are Sports Injuries Classified?

How Are Sprain and Strain Injuries Classified?

No one doubts the benefits of regular structured exercise: elevated cardiovascular fitness; improved muscular strength; and increased flexibility all contribute to an enhanced quality of life. However, one of the very few drawbacks of exercise is an increased susceptibility to sports injury.

While sport and exercise participation rates are increasing, which is a good thing; injury rates are also on the rise. In fact the U.S. Consumer Product Safety Commission estimates that, *"between 1991 and 1998, golf and swimming injuries increased 110 percent; ice hockey and weightlifting injuries, 75 percent; soccer injuries, 55 percent; bicycling, 45 percent; volleyball, 44 percent; and football 43 percent."*

What Constitutes a Sports Injury?

While physical injury generally can be defined as any stress on the body that prevents the organism from functioning properly and results in the body employing a process of repair. A sports injury can be further defined as any kind of injury, pain or physical damage that occurs as a result of sport, exercise or physical activity.

Although the term sports injury can be used to define any injury sustained as a result of sport, it is most commonly used for injuries that affect the musculo-skeletal system, which includes the muscles, bones, tendons, cartilage and associated tissues.

More serious injuries, such as head, neck and spinal cord trauma, are usually considered separate to common sports injuries like sprains, strains, fractures and contusions.

What is Affected in a Sports Injury?

Sports injuries are most commonly associated with the musculo-skeletal system, which includes the muscles, bones, joints and their associated tissues, such as ligaments and tendons. Below is a brief explanation of the components that make up the musculo-skeletal system.

Muscles

Muscle is composed of 75% water, 20% protein, and 5% mineral salts, glycogen, and fat. There are three types of muscle: *skeletal, cardiac,* and *smooth.* The type of muscle involved with movement is *skeletal* (also referred to as striated, and voluntary). Skeletal muscles are under *voluntary control,* and attach to, and cover over, the bony skeleton. Major muscles include the quadriceps in the front of the upper legs and the biceps brachii in the front of the upper arm.

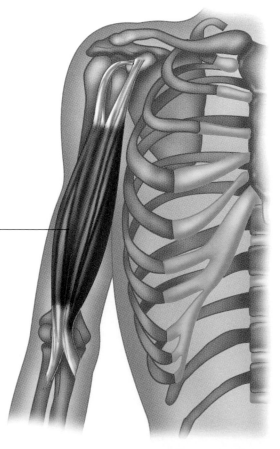

Figure 1.1: Structure of skeletal / striated / voluntary muscle, illustrated with the biceps brachii.

Bones

Bone cells sit in cavities called *lacunae (sing. lacuna)* surrounded by circular layers of very hard matrix that contains calcium salts and larger amounts of collagen fibers. The bones protect internal organs and facilitate movement. Together they form a rigid structure called the *skeleton*. Major bones include the femur in the upper leg and the humerus in the upper arm.

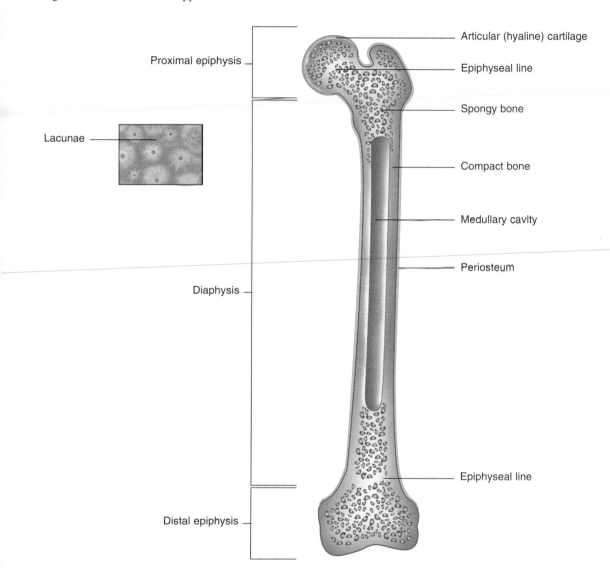

Figure 1.2: Structure of bone, illustrated with the components of a long bone.

Joints

Joints (also called *articulations*) are made up of cartilage, bursa(e), ligaments and tendons, and have two functions: to hold the bones together, and to give the rigid skeleton mobility. *Fibrous joints* have little or no movement, and *cartilaginous joints* are either immovable or slightly movable. Neither has a joint cavity. *Synovial joints* possess a joint cavity that contains *synovial fluid*. They are freely movable, and so are the joints mainly involved with sports injuries. Major synovial joints include the knee, hip, shoulder and elbow.

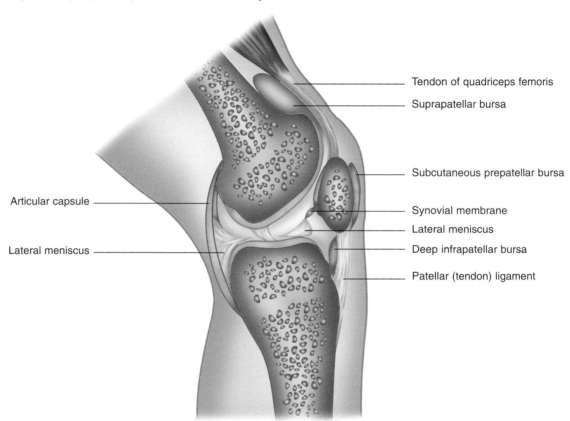

Figure 1.3: The knee joint; right leg, mid-sagittal view.

Cartilage

Cartilage is a specialized, fibrous connective tissue. Examples are: hyaline, fibrocartilage, and elastic. The most important is *hyaline (articular) cartilage*, which is made up of collagen fibers, and water, and covers the articular surface of most joints (see figure 1.2). Cartilage strength is mainly a function of collagen strength, and its main purpose is to provide a smooth surface for the movement of joints and absorb impact and friction when bones bump and rub together.

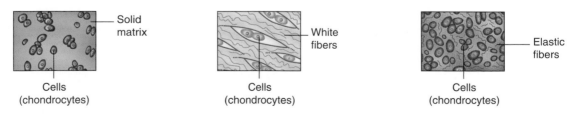

Figure 1.4: Structure of cartilage; a) hyaline cartilage, b) white fibrocartilage, c) yellow elastic cartilage.

Bursae

A bursa (pl. *bursae*) is a small sac, filled with a viscid fluid, and is most commonly found at the point in the joint where the muscle and tendon slide across the bone. The job of a bursa is to reduce friction, and provide smooth movement for the joint (see figure 1.3).

Ligaments

Ligaments are the fibrous connective tissues that connect bone to bone. Composed of dense *regular connective tissue*, ligaments contain more *elastin* than tendons, and so are more *elastic*. Ligaments provide stability for the joints, and with the bones, either allow or limit movement of the limbs (see figure 1.3).

Tendons

Tendons are the fibrous connective tissues that connect muscle to bone. Their collagen fibers are arranged in a parallel pattern, which enables resistance of high, unidirectional tensile loads when the attached muscle contracts. Tendons work together with muscles to exert force on bones and produce movement (see figure 1.3).

Is the Sports Injury Acute or Chronic?

Regardless of where the injury occurs within the body, or the seriousness of the injury, sports injuries are commonly classified in one of two ways: acute or chronic.

Acute injuries

These refer to sports injuries that occur in an instant. Common examples of acute injuries are bone fractures, muscle and tendon strains, ligament sprains and contusions. Acute injuries usually result in pain, swelling, tenderness, weakness and the inability to use or place weight on the injured area.

Chronic injuries

These refer to sports injuries that occur over an extended period of time and are sometimes called *overuse injuries*. Common examples of chronic injuries are tendinitis, bursitis and stress fractures. Chronic injuries, like acute injuries, also result in pain, swelling, tenderness, weakness and the inability to use or place weight on the injured area.

How Are Sports Injuries Classified?

As well as classifying a sports injury as acute or chronic, sports injuries are also classified according to their severity. Injuries are graded into one of three classifications: mild, moderate, or severe.

Mild

A mild sports injury will result in minimal pain and swelling. It will not adversely affect sporting performance and the affected area is neither tender to touch nor deformed in any way.

Moderate

A moderate sports injury will result in some pain and swelling. It will have a limiting affect on sporting performance and the affected area will be mildly tender to touch. Some discoloration at the injury site may also be present.

Severe

A severe sports injury will result in increased pain and swelling. It will not only affect sporting performance, but will also affect normal daily activities. The injury site is usually very tender to touch, and discoloration and deformity are common.

How Are Sprain and Strain Injuries Classified?

The term sprain refers to an injury of the ligaments, as opposed to a strain, which refers to an injury of the muscle or tendon. Remember ligaments attach bone to bone, where as tendons attach muscle to bone.

Injuries to the ligaments, muscles and tendons are usually graded into three categories, and these types of injuries are referred to as: first-, second-, or, third-degree sprains and strains.

First-degree

A first-degree sprain/strain is the least severe. It is the result of some minor stretching of the ligaments, muscles or tendons, and is accompanied by mild pain, some swelling and joint stiffness. There is usually very little loss of joint stability as a result of a first-degree sprain/strain.

Second-degree

A second-degree sprain/strain is the result of both stretching and some tearing of the ligaments, muscles or tendons. There is increased swelling and pain associated with a second-degree sprain/strain, and a moderate loss of stability around the joint.

Third-degree

A third-degree sprain/strain is the most severe of the three. A third-degree sprain/strain is the result of a complete tear or rupture of one or more of the ligaments, muscles or tendons, and will result in massive swelling, severe pain and gross instability.

One interesting point to note about a third-degree sprain/strain is that shortly after the injury, most of the localized pain may disappear. This is a result of the nerve endings being severed, which causes a lack of feeling at the injury site.

Chapter

2

Sports Injury Prevention

Warm-up

Cool-down

The FITT Principle

Overtraining

Fitness and Skill Development

Stretching and Flexibility

Facilities, Rules and Protective Devices

Introduction to Sports Injury Prevention

In a recent article titled *Managing Sports Injuries,* the author estimated that over 27,000 Americans sprain their ankle every day. (And no, that is not a typo, EVERY DAY). On top of this, *Sports Medicine Australia* estimates that 1:17 participants of sport and exercise suffer a sports injury playing their favorite sport. This figure is even higher for contact sports like football and gridiron. However, the truly disturbing fact is that up to 50 percent of these injuries may have been prevented.

If improving sporting performance is the goal, then there is no better way to do that, than by staying injury free. To follow are a number of tips and strategies that will help prevent sports injury. When properly implemented and routinely followed, they have the potential of reducing the incidence of sports injury by up to 50 percent.

Before moving on, please note that any single injury prevention technique discussed in this chapter is just one very important component that assists to reduce the overall risk of injury. The best results are achieved when all the techniques are used in combination with each other. When it comes to sports injury; prevention is better than cure.

Warm-up

The warm-up activities are a crucial part of any exercise or sports training. The importance of a structured warm-up routine should not be underestimated when it comes to the prevention of sports injury.

An effective warm-up has a number of very important key elements. These elements, or parts, should all work together to minimize the likelihood of sports injury from physical activity.

Warming-up prior to any physical activity has a number of benefits, but primarily its main purpose is to prepare the body and mind for more strenuous activity. One of the ways it achieves this is by helping to increase the body's core temperature, while also increasing the body's muscle temperature. Increasing muscle temperature will help to make the muscles loose, supple and pliable.

An effective warm-up also has the effect of increasing both heart rate and respiratory rate. This increases blood flow, which in turn increases the delivery of oxygen and nutrients to the working muscles. All this helps to prepare the muscles, tendons and joints for more strenuous activity.

How Should the Warm-up be Structured?

It is important to start the warm-up routine with the easiest and most gentle activity, building upon each part with more energetic activities until the body is at a physical and mental peak. This is the state in which the body is most prepared for the physical activity to come, and where the likelihood of sports injury has been minimized as much as possible. To achieve these goals, the warm-up should be structured as followed.

There are four key elements, or parts, which should be included to ensure an effective and complete warm-up. They are:

1. The general warm-up;
2. Static stretching;
3. The sports specific warm-up; and,
4. Dynamic stretching.

All four parts are equally important and any one part should not be neglected or thought of as unnecessary. All four elements work together to bring the body and mind to a physical peak, ensuring the athlete is prepared for the activity to come. This process will help ensure the athlete has a minimal risk of sports injury.

1. General warm-up

The general warm-up should consist of light physical activity. The fitness level of the participating athlete should govern both the intensity (how hard) and duration (how long) of the general warm-up. A correct general warm-up for the average person should take about 5–10 minutes and result in a light sweat.

The aim of the general warm-up is to elevate the heart rate and respiratory rate. This in turn increases the blood flow and helps with the transportation of oxygen and nutrients to the working muscles. This also helps to increase the muscle temperature, allowing for a more effective static stretch.

2. Static stretching

Static stretching is a very safe and effective form of stretching. There is a limited threat of injury and it is extremely beneficial for overall flexibility. During this part of the warm-up, static stretching should include all the major muscle groups, and this entire part should last for about five to ten minutes.

Static stretching is performed by placing the body into a position whereby the muscle, (or group of muscles) to be stretched are under tension. Both the opposing muscle group (the muscles behind or in front of the stretched muscle), and the muscles to be stretched are relaxed. Then slowly and cautiously the body is moved to increase the tension of the muscle, or group of muscles to be stretched. At this point the position is held or maintained to allow the muscles and tendons to lengthen.

This second part of an effective warm-up is extremely important, as it helps to lengthen both the muscles and tendons, which in turn allow the limbs a greater range of movement. This is very important in the prevention of muscle and tendon injuries.

The above two elements form the basis, or foundation for a complete and effective warm-up. It is extremely important that these two elements be completed properly before moving onto the next two elements. The proper completion of elements one and two, will now allow for the more specific and vigorous activities necessary for elements three and four.

Recent studies have shown that static stretching may have an adverse affect on muscle contraction speed and therefore impair performance of athletes involved in sports requiring high levels of power and speed. It is for this reason that static stretching is conducted early in the warm-up routine and is always followed by sports specific drills and dynamic stretching.

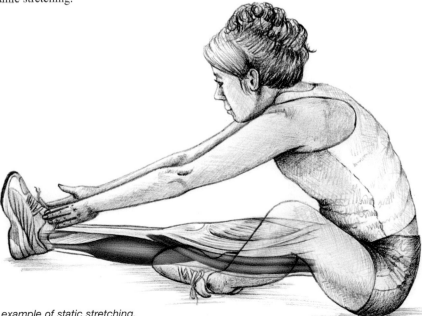

Figure 2.1: An example of static stretching.

3. Sport specific warm-up

With the first two parts of the warm-up carried out thoroughly and correctly, it is now safe to move onto the third part of an effective warm-up. In this part, the athlete is specifically preparing their body for the demands of their particular sport. During this part of the warm-up, more vigorous activity should be employed. Activities should reflect the type of movements and actions that will be required during the sporting event.

4. Dynamic stretching

Finally, a correct warm-up should finish with a series of dynamic stretches. However, this form of stretching carries with it a high risk of injury if used incorrectly. Dynamic stretching is for muscular conditioning as well as flexibility and is really only suited for professional, well-trained, highly conditioned athletes. Dynamic stretching should only be used after a high level of general flexibility has been established.

Dynamic stretching involves a controlled, soft bounce or swinging motion to move a particular body part to the limit of its range of movement. The force of the bounce or swing is gradually increased but should never become radical or uncontrolled.

During this last part of an effective warm-up it is also important to keep the dynamic stretches specific to the athlete's particular sport. This is the final part of the warm-up and should result in the athlete reaching a physical and mental peak. At this point the athlete is most prepared for the rigors of their sport or activity.

The above information forms the basis of a complete and effective warm-up. However, the process described above is somewhat of an ideal or perfect warm-up. This is not always possible or convenient in the real world. Therefore, the individual athlete must become responsible for assessing their own goals and adjusting their warm-up accordingly.

For instance, the time committed to the warm-up should be relative to the level of involvement in the athlete's particular sport. For people just looking to increase their general level of health and fitness, a minimum of 5–10 minutes would be enough. However, if involved in high level competitive sport the athlete will need to dedicate adequate time and effort to a more extensive and complete warm-up.

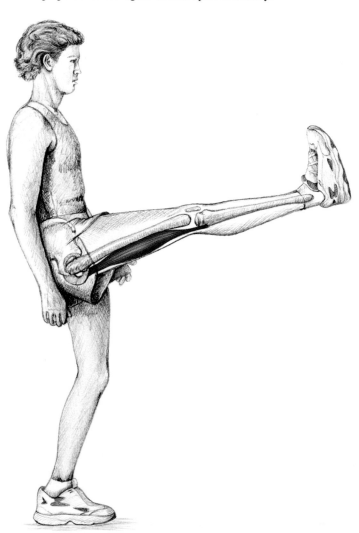

Figure 2.2: An example of dynamic stretching.

Cool-down

Many people dismiss the cool-down as a waste of time, or simply unimportant. In reality the cool-down is just as important as the warm-up, and if you are trying to stay injury free, it is vital.

Although the warm-up and cool-down are just as important as each other, they are important for different reasons. While the main purpose of warming-up is to prepare the body and mind for strenuous activity, cooling-down plays a very different role.

Why Cool-down?

The main aim of the cool-down is to promote recovery and return the body to a pre-exercise, or pre-workout state. During a strenuous workout, the body goes through a number of stressful processes; muscle fibers, tendons and ligaments get damaged, and waste products build up within the body. The cool-down, when performed properly, will assist the body in its repair process, and one area the cool-down will specifically help with is *post-exercise muscle soreness*. Another common term used for post-exercise muscle soreness is *delayed-onset muscle soreness*, or DOMS.

This is the soreness that is usually experienced the day after a tough workout. Most people experience this after having a lay off from exercise, or at the beginning of their sports season. An example of this would be running a 10km fun run or half marathon with very little preparation, and then finding it difficult to walk down steps the next day because the quadriceps muscles are so sore. This discomfort is post-exercise muscle soreness.

This soreness is caused by a number of factors. Firstly, during exercise, tiny tears called microtears develop within the muscle fibers. These microtears cause swelling of the muscle tissues, which in turn put pressure on the nerve endings and result in pain.

Secondly, when exercising, the heart pumps large amounts of blood to the working muscles. This blood carries both oxygen and nutrients that the working muscles need. When the blood reaches the muscles the oxygen and nutrients are used up. Then the force of the contracting (exercising) muscles pushes the blood back to the heart where it is re-oxygenated. However, when the exercise stops, so does the force that pushes the blood back to the heart. This blood, as well as waste products like lactic acid, stays in the muscles, which in turn causes swelling and pain. This process is often referred to as *blood pooling*.

The cool-down helps all of the above by keeping the blood circulating, which in turn helps to prevent blood pooling and also removes waste products from the muscles. This circulating blood also brings with it the oxygen and nutrients needed by the muscles, tendons and ligaments for repair.

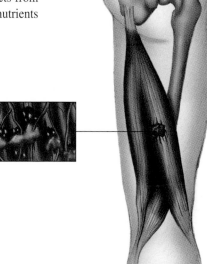

Figure 2.3: Delayed-onset muscle soreness (DOMS).

The Key Parts of an Effective Cool-down

Now that the importance of the cool-down has been established, let us have a look at the structure of an effective cool-down. There are three key elements, or parts, which should be included to ensure an effective and complete cool-down. They are: gentle exercise, stretching, and, re-fuel.

All three elements are equally important and any one part should not be neglected or thought of as unnecessary. They work together to repair and replenish the body after exercise.

To follow are two examples of effective cool-downs. The first is an example of a typical cool-down that would be used by a professional athlete. The second is typical of someone who simply exercises for general health, fitness and fun.

Cool-down Routines for the Professional

* 10–15 minutes of easy exercise. Be sure that the easy exercise resembles the type of exercise that was done during the workout. For example, if the workout involved a lot of running, cool-down with easy jogging or walking.
* Include some deep breathing as part of the easy exercise to help oxygenate the body.
* Follow with about 20–30 minutes of stretching. Static stretching and proprioceptive neuromuscular facilitation (PNF) stretching is best for the cool-down.
* Re-fuel. Both fluid and food are important. Drink plenty of water, plus a good quality sports drink. The best type of food to eat straight after a workout is that which is easily digestible. Fruit is a good example.

Cool-down Routines for the Amateur

* 3–5 minutes of easy exercise. Be sure that the easy exercise resembles the type of exercise that was done during the workout. For example, if the workout involved swimming or cycling, cool-down with a few easy laps of the pool or a slow ride around the block.
* Include some deep breathing as part of the easy exercise to help oxygenate the body.
* Follow with about 5–10 minutes of stretching. Static stretching (see figure 2.1) and PNF stretching (see figure 2.4) is best for the cool-down.
* Re-fuel. Both fluid and food are important. Drink plenty of water, plus a good quality sports drink. The best type of food to eat straight after a workout is that which is easily digestible. Fruit is a good example.

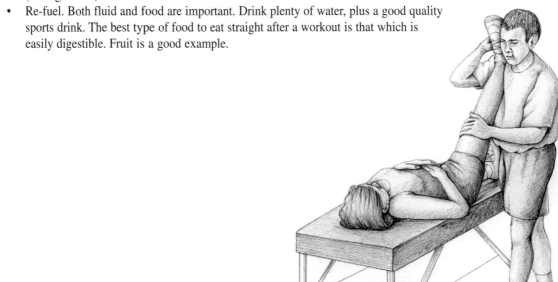

Figure 2.4: An example of PNF stretching

SPORTS INJURY PREVENTION

The FITT Principle

The FITT Principle (or formula) is a great way of monitoring an exercise program. The acronym FITT outlines the key components of an effective exercise program, and the initials stand for:

F: Frequency   **I**: Intensity   **T**: Time   **T**: Type

Frequency

Frequency refers to the frequency of exercise undertaken or how often the athlete exercises. Frequency is a key component of the FITT Principle. Frequency, or the number of times the athlete exercises per week, needs to be adjusted to reflect: the athlete's current fitness level; the time the athlete realistically has available (considering other commitments like family and work); and the specific goals that the athlete has set for themselves.

Intensity

Intensity refers to the intensity of exercise undertaken or how hard the athlete exercises. This is an extremely important aspect of the FITT principle and is probably the hardest factor to monitor. The best way to gauge the intensity of any exercise performed is to monitor heart rate.

There are a couple of ways to monitor heart rate but the best way is to use an exercise heart rate monitor. These can be purchased at most sports stores and consist of an elastic belt that fits around the chest and a wrist watch that displays the exercise heart rate in beats per minute.

Time

Time refers to the time spent exercising or how long the athlete exercises for. The time spent exercising is also an important part of the FITT Principle. The time dedicated to exercise usually depends on the type of exercise undertaken.

For example, it is recommended that to improve cardiovascular fitness we will need at least 20–30 minutes of nonstop exercise. For weight loss, more time is required – at least 40 minutes of moderate weight bearing exercise. However, when talking about the time required for muscular strength improvements, this is often measured as a number of sets and reps (repetitions). A typical recommendation would be three sets of eight reps.

Type

Type refers to the type of exercise undertaken or what kind of exercise the athlete does, and like time, the type of exercise chosen will have a big effect on the results achieved.

For example, if improving cardiovascular fitness is the goal, then exercises like walking, jogging, swimming, bike riding, stair climbing, aerobics and rowing are very effective.

For weight loss, any exercise that uses a majority of our large muscle groups will be effective. To improve muscular strength the best exercises include the use of free weights, machine weights and body weight exercises like push-ups, chin-ups and dips.

How Does All This Relate to Injury Prevention?

The two biggest mistakes people make when designing an exercise program, are to train too hard, and to not include enough variety.

The problem, most commonly, is that people tend to find an exercise they like and very rarely do anything other than that exercise. This can result in long-term, repetitive strain to the same muscle groups, and neglect, or weakening of other muscle groups. This will lead to an unbalanced muscular system, which is a sure-fire recipe for injury.

When using the FITT Principle to design an exercise program, keep the following in mind.

Frequency

After exercise the body goes through a process of rebuilding and repair. It is during this process that the benefits of exercise are forthcoming.

However, if strenuous exercise is conducted on a daily basis (5–6 times a week) the body never has a chance to realize the benefits and gains from the exercise. In this case, what usually happens is that the athlete ends up getting tired or injured, or just quits.

To avoid this scenario, consider more rest and relaxation time, and cut down the frequency of strenuous exercise to only 3–4 times a week.

This may sound strange and a little hard to do at first, because most people have been conditioned into believing that they have to exercise every day, but after a while exercising like this becomes very enjoyable and something that can be looked forward to.

Exercising this way also dramatically reduces the likelihood of injury because the body has more time to repair and heal. Many elite level athletes have seen big improvements in performance when forced to take an extended break. Most never realize they are training too hard, or too often.

Intensity and Time

The key here is variety. Do not get stuck in an exercise rut. Dedicate some of the workouts to long, easy sessions like long walks or light, repetitive weights. While other sessions can be made up of short, high intensity exercises like stair climbing or interval training.

Type

The type of exercise undertaken is also very important. Many people get into a routine of doing the same exercise over and over again. However, if lowering the risk of injury is the goal, do a variety of different exercises. This will help to improve all the major muscle groups and will also help to make the athlete more versatile and well-rounded.

Overtraining

There is a big difference between being just a little tired or on a down-cycle, and being legitimately run down or overtrained. It is important to be able to tell the difference so as to remain injury-free. Nothing will put a stop to improved sporting performance more quickly than not being able to recognize the signs of being legitimately run down and overtrained.

One of the biggest challenges to achieving fitness goals is consistency. If the athlete is repeatedly getting sick, run down and overtrained it becomes very difficult to stay injury free. The following information will help athletes keep the consistency of regular exercise, without overdoing it and becoming sick or injured.

Amateur and professional athletes alike are constantly battling with the problem of overtraining. Being able to juggle just the right amount of training, with enough sleep and rest, and the perfect nutritional diet is not an easy act to master. Throw in a career and a family and it becomes extremely difficult.

What is Overtraining?

Overtraining is the result of giving the body more work or stress than it can handle. Overtraining occurs when a person experiences stress and physical trauma from exercise faster than their body can repair the damage.

This does not happen overnight, or as a result of one or two workouts. In fact, regular exercise is extremely beneficial to general health and fitness, but the athlete must always remember that it is exercise that breaks the body down, while it is the rest and recovery that makes the body strong and healthy. Improvements only occur during the times of rest.

Stress can come from a multitude of sources. It is not just physical stress that causes overtraining. Sure, excessive exercise coupled with inadequate rest will lead to overtraining, but do not forget to consider other stresses, such as family or work commitments. Remember, stress is stress, whether it is a physical, mental or emotional stress, it still has the same effect on the health and wellbeing of the body.

Reading the Signs

At this point in time there are no tests that can be performed to determine whether an athlete is overtrained or not. The athlete cannot go to a local doctor or even a sports medicine laboratory and ask for a test for overtraining. However, while there are no tests for overtraining, there are a number of signs and symptoms that need to be looked out for. These signs and symptoms will act as a warning bell, which will give advanced notice of possible dangers to come.

There are quite a number of signs and symptoms to be on the lookout for, so to make it easier to recognize them, they are grouped below into either, physical or psychological, signs and symptoms.

Suffering from any one or two of the following signs or symptoms does not automatically mean an athlete is suffering from overtraining. However, if a number, say five or six of the following signs and symptoms are recognized, it may be time to take a closer look at the volume and intensity of the current workload.

Physical Signs and Symptoms

- Elevated resting pulse / heart rate;
- Frequent minor infections;
- Increased susceptibility to colds and influenza;
- Increases in minor injuries;
- Chronic muscle soreness or joint pain;
- Exhaustion;
- Lethargy;
- Weight loss;
- Appetite loss;
- Insatiable thirst or dehydration;
- Intolerance to exercise;
- Decreased performance;
- Delayed recovery from exercise.

Psychological Signs and Symptoms

- Fatigued, tired, drained, lack of energy;
- Reduced ability to concentrate;
- Apathy or no motivation;
- Irritability;
- Anxiety;
- Depression;
- Headaches;
- Insomnia;
- Inability to relax;
- Twitchy, fidgety or jittery.

As seen by the number of signs and symptoms, there is a lot to look out for. Generally the most common signs and symptoms to look for are a total loss of motivation in all areas of our life (work or career, health and fitness etc.), plus a feeling of exhaustion. If these two warning signs are present, plus a couple of the other listed signs and symptoms, then it may be time to take a short rest before things get out of hand.

The Answer to the Problem

Let us consider the following example. *We feel run down and totally exhausted. We have no motivation to do anything. We cannot get rid of that niggling knee injury. We are irritable, depressed and have totally lost our appetite.* Sounds like we are overtrained, but what do we do now?

As with most things, prevention is better than cure. To follow are a few measures that can be taken to prevent overtraining.

- Only make small and gradual increases to an exercise program over a period of time.
- Eat a well-balanced, nutritious diet.
- Ensure adequate relaxation and sleep.

- Be prepared to modify the training routine to suit environmental conditions. For example, on a very hot day, go to the pool instead of running on the track.
- Monitor other life stresses and make adjustments to suit.
- Avoid monotonous training by varying exercise routines as much as possible.
- Do not exercise during an illness.
- Be flexible and have some fun with the exercise undertaken.

While prevention should always be the aim, there will be times when overtraining will occur and the following information will help to get the overtrained athlete back on track.

The first priority is to take a rest; anywhere from 3–5 days should do the trick, depending on how severe the overtraining is. During this time the athlete needs to forget about exercise, and the body needs a rest too, so give it one – a physical rest, as well as a mental rest.

Try to get as much sleep and relaxation as possible. Go to bed early and catch a nap whenever possible. Increase the intake of highly nutritious foods and take an extra dose of vitamins and minerals.

After the initial 3–5 days rest the athlete can gradually get back into the normal exercise routine, but start off slowly. Most research states that it is okay to start off with the same intensity and time of exercise but cut back on the frequency. So if the athlete would normally exercise 3–4 times a week, cut that back to only twice a week for the next week or two. After that the athlete should be right to resume the normal exercise regime.

Sometimes it is a good idea to have a rest, like the one outlined above, whether feeling run down or not. It will give both the mind and body a chance to fully recover from any problems that may be building up without the athlete even knowing it. It will also freshen up the mind, give a renewed motivation, and help the athlete look forward to exercise again. Do not underestimate the benefits of a good rest.

Fitness and Skill Development

An individual's physical fitness is made up of a vast number of components. The main components are strength, power, speed, endurance, flexibility, balance, coordination, agility, and skill. Although particular sports require different levels of each fitness component it is essential to plan a regular exercise or training program that covers all of the main components.

A common mistake made by athletes is to excessively focus on the components that are easily recognized within their particular sport, and neglect the others. Although one component may be used more than another, it is important to see each component as only one spoke in the fitness wheel. An imbalance in one component may contribute to sports injury.

For example, football relies heavily on strength and power; however the exclusion of skill drills and flexibility training may lead to serious injury and poor performance. Strength and flexibility are of prime concern to a gymnast but a sound training program would also improve power, speed and endurance.

The same is true for each individual. While some people seem to be naturally strong or flexible, it would be foolish for such a person to completely ignore the other components of physical fitness. This is why such athletes as ironmen and triathletes are often referred to as being totally fit, because their sport demands an even distribution of the components that make up physical fitness.

Defining the appropriate balance is the key to health and fitness success and staying injury free, and may require the assistance of a qualified, professional trainer. To help with the implementation of an exercise or training program, four common training methods are discussed in detail below. They are strength training, circuit training, cross training and plyometic training.

Fitness
Part 1: Strength Training

Strength training has been a part of sports conditioning for many years. It is touted for its effects on speed, strength, agility and muscle mass. Often overlooked though are its benefits for injury prevention.

What is Strength Training?

Strength training is moving the joints through a range of motion against resistance requiring the muscles to expend energy and contract forcefully to move the bones. Strength training can be done using various types of resistance with or without equipment. Strength training is used to strengthen the muscles, tendons, bones and ligaments and to increase muscle mass.

Strength training should be implemented in the conditioning program of all sports, not just strength sports. The increase in speed, strength, agility and muscular endurance will benefit athletes of every sport.

Types of Strength Training

Strength training comes in a variety of formats. The formats are defined by the type of resistance and equipment used.

Machine Weights
Machine strength training includes resistance exercises done using any of the various machines designed to produce resistance. These include machines with weight stacks, hydraulics, resistance rods or bands, and even the use of *Thera-band* or resistance tubing.

The resistance, or weight, may be changed to increase the intensity of the exercise. The range of motion and position of movement is controlled by the machine. The resistance may be constant throughout the movement or may change due to the set-up of the pulley and cam systems. Machines often add a degree of safety but neglect the stabilizer, or helper, muscles in a movement.

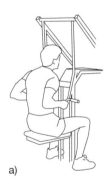
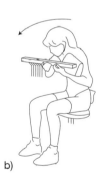
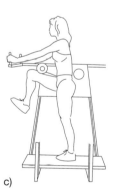

a)   b)   c)

Figure 2.5: Examples of machine weights; a) seated rowing machine, b) abdominal machine, c) multi-hip machine.

Free Weights

Free weight strength training involves using weights that are not fixed in a movement pattern by a machine. These include barbells and dumbbells. Also included in this group are kettlebells, medicine balls, ankle and wrist weights, and weight lifting chains.

The weight used, as with the machines, may be changed to increase the resistance of an exercise. The resistance at different points along the range of motion transfers to different muscles and due to angles may lessen at times. At the lockout of a joint the weight is transferred to the joint as the muscles simply stabilize the joint.

The range of motion and path of movement is not limited so the stabilizing muscles must work to keep the joints in line during the movement. Due to the fact that the movement is not fixed, poor form can become an issue.

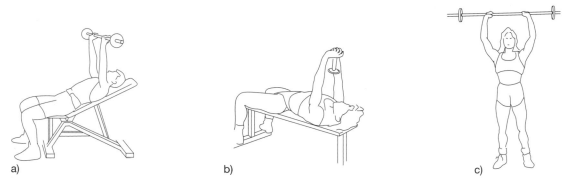

Figure 2.6: Examples of free weights; a) bench press, b) pull overs, c) shoulder press.

Own Body Weight Exercises

Bodyweight exercises involve utilizing the athlete's bodyweight as resistance during the exercise. As with free weights, the range and path of motion is not fixed by a machine. Exercises such as plyometric jumping, push-ups, pull-ups, abdominal exercises, even sprinting and jumping rope, fall into this category.

The weight used in these exercises is constant and only changes when the athlete's body changes. The changes in resistance during the movement are similar to those of free weight exercises.

The range of motion and path of movement does not follow a fixed path so stabilizing muscles come into play. Form is again an issue with these exercises. The inability to change the weight used does limit the effectiveness for some athletes. Larger athletes will be limited in the exercises they can perform and the number of repetitions. Smaller athletes will quickly go beyond the desired repetition range for strength building.

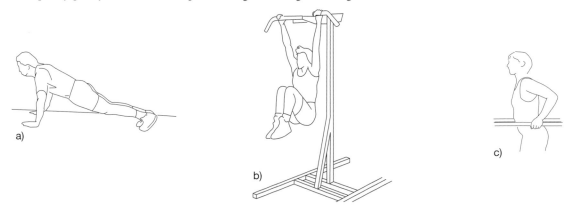

Figure 2.7: Examples of own body weight exercises; a) press-ups, b) hanging leg raise, c) dips.

How Does Strength Training Prevent Injury?

Strength training in athletics is common practice today. The benefits are obvious and the immediate crossover of those benefits to the playing field makes it ideal for off-season conditioning. Injury prevention is one benefit that is often overlooked. Strength training is a very effective tool for injury prevention for a variety of reasons.

Strength training improves the strength of the muscles, tendons, and even the ligaments and bones. The stronger muscles and tendons help to hold the body in proper alignment and protect the bones and joints when moving or under impact. The bones become stronger due to the overload placed on them during training and the ligaments become more flexible and better at absorbing the shock applied to them during dynamic movements.

When an area of the body is used less during an activity it may become weaker than the other areas. This can become a problem when that area (whether a muscle, ligament, joint, or specific bone) is called into play suddenly during an activity. That area cannot handle the sudden stress placed on it and an injury occurs. Strength training, using a balanced program, will eliminate these weak areas and balance the body for the activities it is called to do.

Muscle imbalances are one of the most common causes of injuries in athletics. When one muscle, or muscle group, becomes stronger than its opposing group, the weaker muscles become fatigued quicker and more susceptible to injury. A forceful contraction, near maximal output from the stronger muscle can also cause damage to the weaker opposing muscle due to the inability to counter the force.

Muscle imbalances also affect the joints and bones due to an abnormal pull causing the joint to move in an unnatural pattern. The stronger muscles will cause the joint to pull in that direction causing a stretching of the opposing ligaments and a tightening of the supporting ones. These can lead to chronic pain and an unnatural wearing of the bones. A balanced strength training program will help to counter these effects by strengthening the weaker muscles to balance them with their counterparts.

Precautions for Strength Training

Strength training is a great tool for injury prevention. Becoming injured during strength training obviously defeats this purpose. To avoid injury it is essential that proper form be used in all exercises. Keeping the body in proper alignment while exercising will minimize the injury chances. Starting with light weights or resistance and developing proper form before increasing the resistance is important. When increasing the resistance it is important to do so in small increments and only when the desired number of repetitions can be performed in correct form.

Rest plays a crucial role in the efficiency and safety of a training program. Remember the muscles repair and become stronger during rest, not during the workout. Performing strength training exercises for the same muscle groups without adequate rest between training sessions can lead to overtraining. Overtraining will result in the muscles being unable to repair properly and not being ready for additional work. This can lead to acute or chronic injuries.

Fitness
Part 2: Circuit Training

Circuit training routines are a favorite training session for many coaches and athletes. Circuit training can be used as part of injury rehabilitation programs, for conditioning elite level athletes, or to help with weight loss. Circuits can be used for just about everything.

An exceptional sports coach by the name of Col Stewart is a big fan of circuit training routines. Col is one of those rare coaches who can take just about any sport and devise a specific training program that always produces outstanding improvements for his athletes.

Col's circuit training routines are largely responsible for the success of many of his world champion athletes. Including his son, Miles Stewart (World Champion Triathlete), Mick Doohan (World 500cc Motorcycle Champion), and countless others from sports as diverse as roller-skating, squash, and cycling. Many other coaches are also impressed by circuit training and use it regularly.

Brian Mackenzie from Sports Coach says, *"Circuit training is an excellent way to simultaneously improve mobility, strength and stamina."*

Workouts for Women state, *"Circuit training is one of the best methods of exercising as it provides excellent all round fitness, tone, strength, and a reduction of weight and inches. In short, maximum results in minimum time."*

And another site referred to circuit training as, *"An ideal way to build versatility, overall strength and fitness, as well as to consolidate the mastery of a wide variety of physical skills."*

What is Circuit Training?

Circuit training consists of a consecutive series of timed exercises performed one after the other with varying amounts of rest between each exercise.

For example, a simple circuit training routine might consist of push-ups, sit-ups, squats, chin-ups and lunges. The routine might be structured as follows, and could be continually repeated as many times as is necessary.

- Do as many push-ups as we can in 30 seconds, then rest for 30 seconds.
- Do as many squats as we can in 30 seconds, then rest for 30 seconds.
- Do as many sit-ups as we can in 30 seconds, then rest for 30 seconds.
- Do as many lunges as we can in 30 seconds, then rest for 30 seconds.
- Do as many chin-ups as we can in 30 seconds, then rest for 30 seconds.

What Makes Circuit Training So Good?

The quick pace and constant changing nature of circuit training places a unique type of stress on the body, which differs from normal exercise activities, like weight training and aerobic exercise.

The demands of circuit training prepare the body in a very even, all-round manner. Circuit training is an exceptional form of exercise to aid in the prevention of injury and is one of the best ways to condition the entire body and mind.

There are many other reasons why circuit training is a fantastic form of exercise and what most of these reasons come down to is flexibility. In other words, circuit training is totally customizable to the specific requirements of the individual.

- Circuit training can be totally personalized. Whether a beginner, or elite athlete, circuit training routines can be modified to give the best possible results.

- A circuit training routine can be modified to give the athlete exactly what they want. Whether an all-over body workout, or just working on a specific body area, or working on a particular aspect of the chosen sport, this can all be accommodated.
- It is easy to change the focus of the circuit training routine to emphasize strength, endurance, agility, speed, skill development, weight loss, or any other aspect of fitness that is important to the individual.
- Circuit training is time efficient. No wasted time in between sets. It is maximum results in minimum time.
- Circuit training can be done just about anywhere. Circuit training is a favorite form of exercise for the British Royal Marine Commandos because they spend a lot of time on large ships. The confined spaces means that circuit training is sometimes the only form of exercise available to them.
- No expensive equipment is needed; not even a gym membership. It is just as easy to put together a great circuit training routine at home or in a park. By using some imagination, it is easy to devise all sorts of exercises using things like chairs and tables, and even children's outdoor play equipment like swings and monkey bars.
- Another reason why circuit training is so popular is that it is great fun to do in pairs or groups. Half the group performs the exercises, while the other half rests and motivates the exercising members of the group.

Types of Circuit Training

As mentioned before, circuit training can be totally customized, which means there are an unlimited number of different ways to structure a circuit training routine. Here are a few examples of the different types available.

Timed Circuit
This type of circuit involves working to a set time period for both rest and exercise intervals. For example, a typical timed circuit might involve 30 seconds of exercise and 30 seconds of rest in between each exercise.

Competition Circuit
This is similar to a timed circuit but each individual pushes himself or herself to see how many repetitions can be done in the set time period. For example, complete 12 push-ups in 30 seconds. The idea is to keep the time period the same, but try to increase the number of repetitions done in the set time period.

Repetition Circuit
This type of circuit is great when working with large groups of people who have different levels of fitness and ability. The idea is that the fittest group might do 20 repetitions of each exercise; the intermediate group might only do 15 repetitions; while the beginners might only do 10 repetitions of each exercise.

Sport Specific or Running Circuit
This type of circuit is best done outside or in a large, open area. Choose exercises that are specific to the participants' sport, or emphasize an aspect of the sport that needs improvement. Then instead of simply resting between exercises, run easy for 200 or 400 meters.

Some Important Precautions

Circuit training is a fantastic form of exercise. However, the most common problem is that people tend to get over excited, because of the timed nature of the exercises, and push themselves harder than they normally would. This tends to result in sore muscles and joints, and an increased likelihood of injury. Below are two precautions to take into consideration.

Level of Fitness

If the athlete has never done any sort of circuit training before, even if they are considered quite fit, start off slowly. The nature of circuit training is quite different to any other form of exercise. It places different demands on the body and mind, and if the athlete is not used to it, it will take a few sessions for the body to adapt to this new form of training.

Warm-up and Cool-down

Do not ever start a circuit training routine without a thorough warm-up that includes stretching. As mentioned previously, circuit training is very different from other forms of exercise. The body must be prepared for circuit training before starting a session.

Fitness
Part 3: Cross Training

Cross training, although it has been used for years, is relatively new as a training concept. Athletes have been forced to use exercises outside their sport for conditioning for many reasons, including: weather, seasonal change, facility and equipment availability, and injuries. These athletes were cross training whether they knew it or not. The benefits of cross training are beginning to get more press and one of those is injury prevention.

What is Cross Training?

Cross training is the use of various activities to achieve overall conditioning. Cross training uses activities outside the normal drills and exercises commonly associated with a sport. The exercises provide a break from the normal impact of training in a particular sport, thereby giving the muscles, tendons, bones, joints and ligaments a brief break. These exercises target the muscles from a different angle or resistance and work to balance an athlete. Cross training is an effective way of resting the body from the normal sport-specific activities while maintaining conditioning.

Any exercise or activity can be used for cross training if it is not a skill associated with that particular sport. Weight training is a commonly used cross training tool. Swimming, cycling, running, and even skiing are activities used for cross training. Plyometrics are becoming popular again as cross training tools.

Critics of Cross Training

Cross training does help achieve balance in the muscles due to working them from various angles and in different positions. Cross training does not however, develop skills specific to the sport or sport-specific conditioning. A football player who jogs three to five miles all summer and lifts weights will still not be in *football shape* when the preseason starts. Cross training cannot be used as the sole conditioning tool. Sport specific conditioning and skill training is still required.

High impact sports such as basketball, gymnastics, football or running cause a lot of jarring on the skeletal system. Cross training can help limit the jarring but some sport-specific impact is necessary to condition athletes for their activity. A runner who runs in water as their only conditioning routine may develop shin splints and other injuries when they are required to run on hard surfaces for races or training. Their body is not conditioned to the forces it is subjected to and will react accordingly.

Jumping into an intense cross training schedule without progressing into it properly can also lead to problems. It is important to progressively increase the intensity, duration and frequency in small increments.

Cross Training Examples

Cross training can take many forms. The key to a successful cross training program is that it must address the same energy systems used in the sport and must allow a break from sport-specific activities. Training the same major muscle groups, but in a different way keeps the athlete conditioned but helps prevent overuse injuries.

- A cyclist may use swimming to build upper body strength and to maintain cardiovascular endurance. They may use cross-country skiing to maintain leg strength and endurance when snow and ice eliminate biking time.
- Swimmers may use free weight training to develop and maintain strength levels. They may incorporate rock climbing to keep upper body strength and endurance up.
- Runners may use mountain biking to target the legs from a slightly different approach. They can use deep water running to lessen the impact while still maintaining a conditioning schedule.
- A shot putter may use Olympic weightlifting exercises to build overall explosiveness. They may use plyometrics and sprinting to develop the needed explosiveness in the hips and legs.

How Does Cross Training Prevent Injury?

Cross training is an important tool in the injury prevention program of athletes. Cross training allows coaches and athletes the opportunity to train hard all year round without running the risk of overtraining or overuse injuries. The simple process of changing the type of training changes the stress on the body.

Cross training gives the muscles used in the primary sport a break from the normal stresses put on them each day. The muscles may still be worked, even intensely, but without the normal impact or from a different angle. This allows the muscles to recover from the wear and tear built up over a season. This active rest is a much better recovery tool than total rest and forces the body to adapt to different stimuli.

Cross training also helps to reduce or reverse muscle imbalances in the body. A pitcher in baseball may develop an imbalance laterally between the two sides of the body as well as in the shoulder girdle of the throwing arm. Thousands of pitches over a season will cause the muscles directly involved in throwing to become stronger while supporting muscles and those unaffected by throwing will become weaker without training. Cross training can help balance the strength in the muscles on both sides as well as the stabilizing muscles. This balancing of strength and flexibility helps to prevent one muscle group, due to a strength imbalance, from pulling the body out of natural alignment. It also prevents muscle pulls and tears caused by one muscle exerting more force than the opposing group can counter.

Precautions for Cross Training

Whenever starting a new activity it is important to get instruction in the proper techniques and safety measures. Ocean kayaking can be a great cross training activity for tennis players to develop and maintain upper body endurance but without instruction on proper techniques it can be dangerous.

Equipment used for cross training activities should be fitted properly and designed for the activity. Unsafe or ill-fitted equipment can lead to injury.

Cross training is a great way to avoid overuse injuries and overtraining. Unfortunately, these same pitfalls can be an issue in a cross training program. Varying workouts, adequate rest between workouts, use of proper form and gradual increasing of resistance are important in any program. Many athletes simply add cross training to their current program rather than substituting. This leads to overtraining and the opposite of the injury prevention goal.

SPORTS INJURY PREVENTION

Fitness
Part 4: Plyometric Training

The previous three sections looked at three very good training techniques to help develop and condition athletic ability, which in-turn will help to prevent sports injury. This section will build on the last three techniques by discussing a slightly more advanced form of athletic conditioning called plyometrics.

What are Plyometric Exercises?

In the simplest of terms, plyometrics are exercises that involve a jumping movement. For example, side to side jumping, bounding, jumping rope, punchbag push, hopping, lunges, trunk curl and throw, jump squats, and clap push-ups are all examples of plyometric exercises.

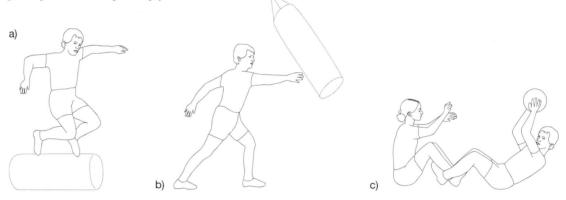

Figure 2.8: Examples of plyometric exercises; a) side to side jumping, b) punchbag push, c) trunk curl and throw.

However, for a more detailed definition some background information about muscle contractions is needed. Muscles contract in one of three ways:

1. Eccentric Muscle Contraction

An eccentric muscle contraction occurs when the muscle contracts and lengthens at the same time. An example of an eccentric muscle contraction is lowering an object held in the hand down to your side. The biceps brachii (upper arm) muscle contracts eccentrically to enable controlled lowering of the arm.

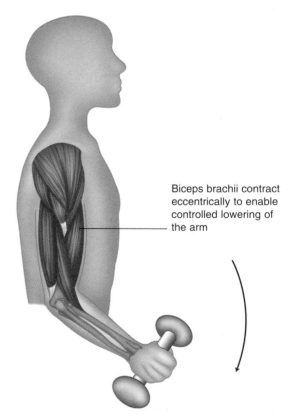

Biceps brachii contract eccentrically to enable controlled lowering of the arm

Figure 2.9: Eccentric muscle contraction.

2. Concentric Muscle Contraction

A concentric muscle contraction occurs when the muscle contracts and shortens at the same time. An example of a concentric muscle contraction is lifting the body up into a chin-up position. The biceps brachii muscle contracts and shortens as the body is raised up to the chin-up bar.

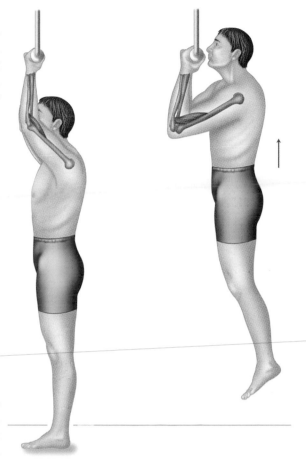

Figure 2.10: Concentric muscle contraction.

3. Isometric Muscle Contraction

An isometric muscle contraction occurs when the muscle contracts, but does not change in length. An example of an isometric muscle contraction is holding a heavy object in the hand with the elbow held stationary and bent at 90 degrees. The biceps brachii muscle contracts, but does not change in length because the body is not moving up or down.

Getting back to the formal definition; a plyometric exercise is an exercise in which an eccentric muscle contraction is quickly followed by a concentric muscle contraction. In other words, when a muscle is rapidly contracted and lengthened, and then immediately followed with a further contraction and shortening, this is a plyometric exercise. This process of contract-lengthen, contract-shorten is often referred to as the *stretch-shortening cycle*.

Here is another example of a plyometric exercise. Consider the simple act of jumping off a step, landing on the ground with both feet, and then jumping forward; all done in one swift movement.

When jumping off the step and landing on the ground, the muscles in the legs contract eccentrically to slow the body down. Thus, when jumping forward, the muscles contract concentrically to spring off the ground. This is a classic example of a plyometric exercise.

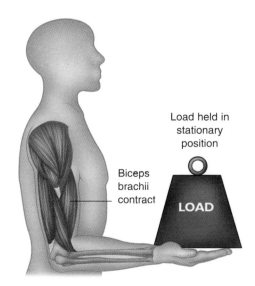

Load held in stationary position

Biceps brachii contract

LOAD

Figure 2.11: Isometric muscle contraction.

Why are Plyometric Exercises Important for Injury Prevention?

Athletes to develop power for their chosen sport often use plyometrics, and a lot has been written about how to accomplish this. However, few people realize how important plyometrics can be in aiding injury prevention.

Essentially, plyometric exercises force the muscle to contract rapidly from a full stretch position. This is the position in which muscles tend to be at their weakest. By conditioning the muscle at its weakest point, (full stretch) it is better prepared to handle this type of stress in a real or game environment.

Why are Plyometric Exercises Important for Injury Rehabilitation?

Most injury rehabilitation programs fail to realize that an eccentric muscle contraction can be up to three times more forceful than a concentric muscle contraction. This is why plyometric exercises are important in the final stage of rehabilitation, to condition the muscles to handle the added strain of eccentric contractions.

Neglecting this final stage of the rehabilitation process can often lead to re-injury, because the muscles have not been conditioned to cope with the added force of eccentric muscle contractions.

Caution, Caution, Caution!

Plyometrics are NOT for everyone. Plyometric exercises are not for the amateur and they are not for the weekend warrior. They are an advanced form of athletic conditioning and can place a massive strain on unconditioned muscles, joints and bones.

Plyometric exercises should only be used by well-conditioned athletes and preferably under the supervision of a professional sports coach. When adding plyometric exercises to a regular training routine, please take careful note of the following precautions.

- Children or teenagers who are still growing should not use intense, repetitive plyometric exercises.
- A solid base of muscular strength and endurance should be developed before starting a plyometrics program. In fact Better-Body.com recommends; *"It is a good rule of thumb that before we start using any plyometric exercises we should be able to squat at least 1.5 times our own body weight, and then focus on developing core strength."*
- A thorough warm-up is essential to ensure the athlete is ready for the intensity of plyometric exercises.
- Do not perform plyometric exercises on concrete, asphalt or other hard surfaces. Grass is one of the best surfaces for plyometric exercises.
- Technique is important. As soon as form deteriorates or the athlete feels tired, back off.
- Do not overdo it. Plyometrics are very intense. Allow plenty of rest between sessions, and do not perform plyometric exercises two days in a row.

Stretching and Flexibility
Part 1: How Does Stretching Prevent Sports Injury?

Stretching is a simple and effective activity that helps to enhance athletic performance, decrease the likelihood of injury and minimize muscle soreness. But how specifically does stretching prevent sports injury?

Improved Range of Movement

By placing particular parts of the body in certain positions, we are able to increase the length of our muscles. As a result of this, a reduction in general muscle tension is achieved and our normal range of movement is increased.

By increasing our range of movement we are increasing the distance our limbs can move before damage occurs to the muscles and tendons. For example, the muscles and tendons in the back of our legs are put under great strain when kicking a football. Therefore, the more flexible and pliable those muscles are, the further our leg can travel forward before a strain or injury occurs to them.

The benefits of an extended range of movement include: increased comfort; a greater ability to move freely; and a lessening of our susceptibility to muscle and tendon strain injuries.

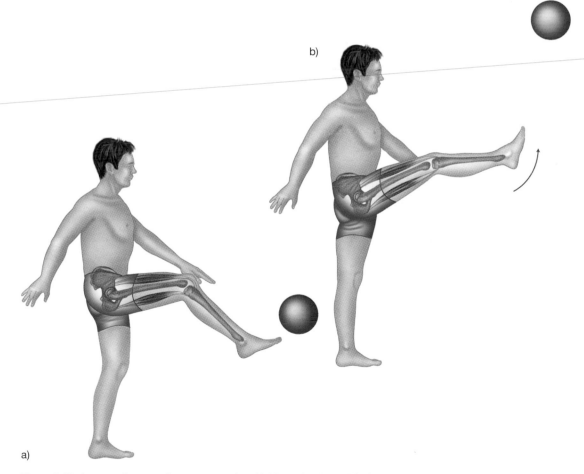

b)

a)

Figure 2.12: Improved range of movement when kicking a football; a) limited range of movement, b) improved range of movement after conditioning.

Reduced Post-exercise Muscle Soreness

We have all experienced what happens when we go for a run or to the gym for the first time in a few months. The following day our muscles are tight, sore, stiff and it is usually hard to even walk down a flight of stairs. The soreness that usually accompanies strenuous physical activity is often referred to as *post-exercise muscle soreness* (see figure 2.3). This soreness is the result of micro tears, (minute tears within the muscle fibers), blood pooling and accumulated waste products, such as lactic acid. Stretching, as part of an effective cool-down, helps to alleviate this soreness by lengthening the individual muscle fibers, increasing blood circulation, and removing waste products.

Reduced Fatigue

Fatigue is a major problem for everyone, especially those who exercise. It results in a decrease in both physical and mental performance. Increased flexibility through stretching can help prevent the effects of fatigue by taking pressure off the working muscles, (the *agonist*). For every muscle in the body there is an opposite or opposing muscle, (the *antagonist*). If the opposing muscles are more flexible, the working muscles do not have to exert as much force against the opposing muscles. Therefore each movement of the working muscles actually takes less effort.

Added Benefits

Along with the benefits listed above, a regular stretching program will also help to improve posture, develop body awareness, improve coordination, promote circulation, increase energy, and, improve relaxation and stress relief.

Part 2: The Rules for Safe Stretching

As with most activities there are rules and guidelines to ensure that they are safe. Stretching is no exception. Stretching can be extremely dangerous and harmful if done incorrectly. It is vitally important that the following rules be adhered to, both for safety and for maximizing the potential benefits of stretching.

There is often confusion and concerns about which stretches are good and which stretches are bad. In most cases someone has told the inquirer that they should not do this stretch or that stretch, or that this is a good stretch and this is a bad stretch.

Are there only good stretches and bad stretches? Is there no middle ground? And if there are only good and bad stretches, how do we decide which ones are good and which ones are bad? Let us put an end to the confusion once and for all...

There is no such thing as a good or bad stretch!

Just as there are no good or bad exercises, there are no good or bad stretches; only what is appropriate for the specific requirements of the individual. So a stretch that is perfectly okay for one person may not be okay for someone else.

Let me use an example. A person with a shoulder injury would not be expected to do push-ups or freestyle swimming, but that does not mean that these are bad exercises. Now, consider the same scenario from a stretching point of view. That same person should avoid shoulder stretches, but that does not mean that all shoulder stretches are bad.

The stretch itself is neither good nor bad. It is the way the stretch is performed and whom it is being performed on that makes stretching either effective and safe, or ineffective and harmful. To place a particular stretch into a category of good or bad is foolish and dangerous. To label a stretch as good gives people the impression that they can do that stretch whenever and however they want and it will not cause them any problems.

The specific requirements of the individual are what are important!

Remember, stretches are neither good nor bad. However, when choosing a stretch there are a number of *precautions* and *checks* we need to perform before giving that stretch the okay.

1. Firstly, make a general review of the individual. Are they healthy and physically active, or have they been leading a sedentary lifestyle for the past five years? Are they a professional athlete? Are they recovering from a serious injury? Do they have aches, pains or muscle and joint stiffness in any area of their body?

2. Secondly, make a specific review of the area, or muscle group to be stretched. Are the muscles healthy? Is there any damage to the joints, ligaments, tendons, etc.? Has the area been injured recently, or is it still recovering from an injury?

If the muscle group being stretched is not 100% healthy, avoid stretching this area altogether. Work on recovery and rehabilitation before moving onto specific stretching exercises. If however, the individual is healthy and the area to be stretched is free from injury, then apply the following to all stretches.

Warm-up Prior to Stretching

This first rule is often overlooked and can lead to serious injury if not performed effectively. Trying to stretch muscles that have not been warmed is like trying to stretch old, dry rubber bands: they may snap.

Warming-up prior to stretching does a number of beneficial things, but primarily its purpose is to prepare the body and mind for more strenuous activity. One of the ways it achieves this is by helping to increase the body's core temperature while also increasing the body's muscle temperature. By increasing muscle temperature we are helping to make the muscles loose, supple and pliable. This is essential to ensure the maximum benefit is gained from our stretching.

The correct warm-up also has the effect of increasing both our heart rate and respiratory rate. This increases blood flow, which in turn increases the delivery of oxygen and nutrients to the working muscles. All this helps to prepare the muscles for stretching.

A correct warm-up should consist of light physical activity. The fitness level of the participating athlete should govern both the intensity and duration of the warm-up, although a correct warm-up for most people should take about ten minutes, and result in a light sweat.

Stretch Before and After Exercise

The question often arises, *"should I stretch before or after exercise?"* This is not an either/or situation, as both are essential. It is no good stretching after exercise and counting that as the pre-exercise stretch for next time. Stretching after exercise has a totally different purpose to stretching before exercise. The two are not the same.

The purpose of stretching before exercise is to help prevent injury. Stretching does this by lengthening the muscles and tendons, which in turn increases our range of movement. This ensures that we are able to move freely without restriction or injury occurring.

However, stretching after exercise has a very different role. Its purpose is primarily to aid in the repair and recovery of the muscles and tendons. By lengthening the muscles and tendons, stretching helps to prevent tight muscles and delayed muscle soreness that usually accompanies strenuous exercise.

After exercise our stretching should be done as part of a cool-down. The cool-down will vary depending on the duration and intensity of exercise undertaken, but will usually consist of 5–10 minutes of very light physical activity and be followed by 5–10 minutes of static stretching exercises.

An effective cool-down involving light physical activity and stretching, will help to rid waste products from the muscles, prevent blood pooling, and promote the delivery of oxygen and nutrients to the muscles. All this assists in returning the body to a pre-exercise level, thus aiding the recovery process.

Stretch All Major Muscles and Their Opposing Muscle Groups

When stretching, it is vitally important that we pay attention to all the major muscle groups in the body. Just because a particular sport may place a lot of emphasis on the legs for example, does not mean that one can neglect the muscles of the upper body in a stretching routine.

All the muscles play an important part in any physical activity, not just a select few. Muscles in the upper body for example, are extremely important in any running sport. They play a vital role in the stability and balance of the body during the running motion. Therefore it is important to keep them both flexible and supple.

Every muscle in the body has an opposing muscle that acts against it. For example, the muscles in the front of the leg (the quadriceps) are opposed by the muscles in the back of the leg (the hamstrings). These two groups of muscles provide a resistance to each other to balance the body. If one of these groups of muscles becomes stronger or more flexible than the other group, it is likely to lead to imbalances that can result in injury or postural problems.

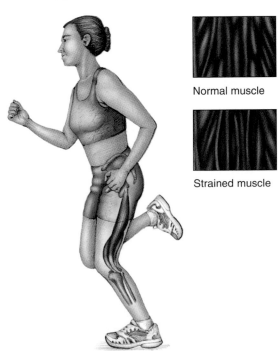

Normal muscle

Strained muscle

Figure 2.13: A hamstring tear whilst running, due to tightness of the muscle.

For example, hamstring tears are a common injury in most running sports. They are often caused by strong quadriceps and weak, inflexible hamstrings. This imbalance puts a great deal of pressure on the hamstrings and can result in a muscle tear or strain.

Stretch Gently and Slowly

Stretching gently and slowly helps to relax our muscles, which in turn makes stretching more pleasurable and beneficial. This will also help to avoid muscle tears and strains that can be caused by rapid, jerky movements.

Stretch ONLY to the Point of Tension

Stretching is NOT an activity that is meant to be painful; it should be pleasurable, relaxing and very beneficial. Although many people believe that to get the most from their stretching they need to be in constant pain. This is one of the greatest mistakes we can make when stretching. Let me explain why.

When the muscles are stretched to the point of pain, the body employs a defense mechanism called the stretch reflex. This is the body's safety measure to prevent serious damage occurring to the muscles, tendons and joints. The stretch reflex protects the muscles and tendons by contracting them, thereby preventing them from being stretched.

So to avoid the stretch reflex, avoid pain. Never push the stretch beyond what is comfortable. Only stretch to the point where tension can be felt in the muscles. This way, injury will be avoided and the maximum benefits from stretching will be achieved.

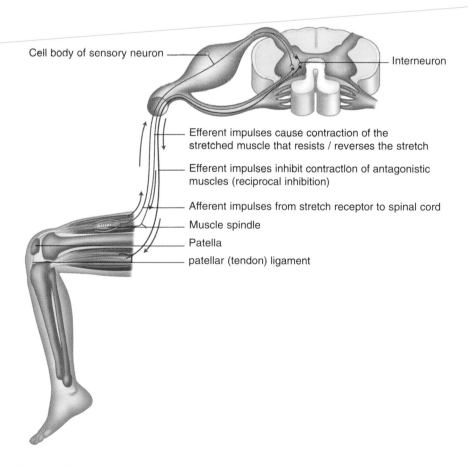

Cell body of sensory neuron

Interneuron

Efferent impulses cause contraction of the stretched muscle that resists / reverses the stretch

Efferent impulses inhibit contraction of antagonistic muscles (reciprocal inhibition)

Afferent impulses from stretch receptor to spinal cord

Muscle spindle

Patella

patellar (tendon) ligament

Figure 2.14: The stretch reflex arc.

Breathe Slowly and Easily While Stretching

Many people unconsciously hold their breath while stretching. This causes tension in our muscles, which in turn makes it very difficult to stretch. To avoid this, remember to breathe slowly and deeply during all stretching exercises. This helps to relax our muscles, promotes blood flow and increases the delivery of oxygen and nutrients to our muscles.

An Example
By taking a look at one of the most controversial stretches ever performed, we can see how the above rules are applied.

The stretch pictured below causes many a person to go into complete meltdown. It has a reputation as a dangerous, bad stretch and should be avoided at all costs.

So why is it that at every Olympic Games, Commonwealth Games and World Championships, sprinters can be seen doing this stretch before their events? Let us apply the above checks to find out.

Firstly, consider the person performing the stretch. Are they healthy, fit and physically active? If not, this is not a stretch they should be doing. Are they elderly, overweight or unfit? Are they young and still growing? Do they lead a sedentary lifestyle? If so, they should avoid this stretch! This first consideration alone would prohibit 50% of the population from doing this stretch.

Secondly, review the area to be stretched. This stretch obviously puts a large strain on the muscles of the hamstrings and lower back. So if our hamstrings or lower back are not 100% healthy, do not perform this stretch.

This second consideration would probably rule out another 25%, which means this stretch is only suitable for about 25% of the population: or, the well-trained, physically fit, injury free athlete.

Then apply the six precautions above and the well-trained, physically fit, injury free athlete can perform this stretch safely and effectively.

Remember, the stretch itself is neither good, nor bad. It is the way the stretch is performed and by whom it is being performed that makes stretching either effective and safe, or ineffective and harmful.

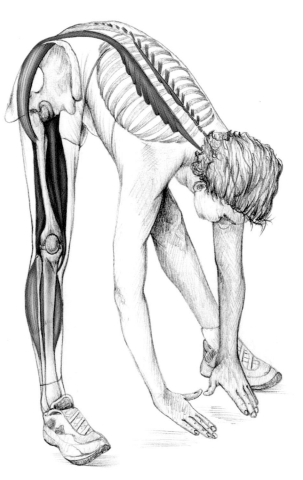

Figure 2.15: A controversial stretch?

Part 3: How to Stretch Properly

When to Stretch

Stretching needs to be as important as the rest of our training. If we are involved in any competitive type of sport or exercise then it is crucial that we make time for specific stretching workouts. Set time aside to work on particular areas that are tight or stiff. The more involved and committed we are to our exercise and fitness, the more time and effort we will need to commit to stretching.

As discussed earlier it is important to stretch both before and after exercise. But when else should we stretch and what type of stretching is best for a particular purpose?

Choosing the right type of stretching for the right purpose will make a big difference to the effectiveness of our flexibility program. To follow are some suggestions for when to use the different types of stretches.

For warming-up, dynamic stretching is the most effective, while for cooling-down, static, passive and PNF stretching is best. For improving range of movement, try PNF and active isolated stretching, and for rehabilitation, a combination of PNF, isometric and active stretching will give the best results.

So when else should we stretch? Stretch periodically throughout the entire day. It is a great way to keep loose and to help ease the stress of everyday life. One of the most productive ways to utilize our time is to stretch while we are watching television. Start with five minutes of marching or jogging on the spot then take a seat on the floor in front of the television and start stretching.

Competition is a time when great demands are placed on the body; therefore it is vitally important that we are in peak physical condition. Our flexibility should be at its best just before competition. Too many injuries are caused by the sudden exertion that is needed for any sort of competitive sport. Get strict on stretching before competition.

Hold, Count, Repeat

For how long should I hold each stretch? How often should I stretch? For how long should I stretch?
These are the most commonly asked questions when discussing the topic of stretching. Although there are conflicting responses to these questions, it is my professional opinion that through a study of research literature and personal experience, I believe what follows is currently the most correct and beneficial information.

The question that causes the most conflict is: *"For how long should I hold each stretch?"* Some text will tell us that as little as ten seconds is enough. This is a bare minimum. Ten seconds is only just enough time for the muscles to relax and start to lengthen. For any real benefit to our flexibility we should hold each stretch for at least twenty to thirty seconds.

The time we commit to our stretching will be relative to our level of involvement in our particular sport. So, for people looking to increase their general level of health and fitness, a minimum of about twenty seconds will be enough. However, if we are involved in high-level competitive sport we need to hold each stretch for at least thirty seconds and start to extend that to sixty seconds and beyond.

"How often should I stretch?" This same principle of adjusting our level of commitment to our level of involvement in our sport applies to the number of times we should stretch each muscle group. For example, the beginner should stretch each muscle group two to three times. However, if we are involved at a more advanced level in our sport we should stretch each muscle group three to five times.

"For how long should I stretch?" The same principle applies. For the beginner, about five to ten minutes is enough, and for the professional athlete, anything up to two hours. If we feel that we are somewhere between the beginner and the professional adjust the time we spend stretching accordingly.

Please do not be impatient with stretching. Nobody can get fit in a couple of weeks so do not expect miracles from a stretching routine. Looking long-term, some muscles groups may need a minimum of three months of intense stretching to see any real improvement. So stick with it, it is well worth the effort.

Sequence

When starting a stretching program it is a good idea to start with a general range of stretches for the entire body, instead of just a select few. The idea of this is to reduce overall muscle tension and to increase the mobility of our joints and limbs.

The next step should be to increase overall flexibility by starting to extend the muscles and tendons beyond their normal range of movement. Following this, work on specific areas that are tight or important for our particular sport. Remember, all this takes time. This sequence of stretches may take up to three months for us to see real improvement, especially if we have no background in agility based activities or are heavily muscled.

No data exists on what order we should do our stretches in. However, it is recommended that we start with sitting stretches, because there is less chance of injury while sitting, before moving on to standing stretches. To make it easier we may want to start with the ankles and move up to the neck or vice-versa. It really does not matter as long as we cover all the major muscle groups and their opposing muscles.

Once we have advanced beyond improving our overall flexibility and are working on improving the range of movement of specific muscles, or muscle groups, it is important to isolate those muscles during our stretching routines. To do this, concentrate on only one muscle group at a time. For example, instead of trying to stretch both hamstrings at the same time, concentrate on only one at a time. Stretching this way will help to reduce the resistance from other supporting muscle groups.

Posture

Posture, or alignment, while stretching is one of the most neglected aspects of flexibility training. It is important to be aware of how crucial it can be to the overall benefits of our stretching. Bad posture and incorrect technique can cause imbalances in the muscles that can lead to injury. While proper posture will ensure that the targeted muscle group receives the best possible stretch.

In many instances a major muscle group can be made up of a number of different muscles. If our posture is sloppy or incorrect certain stretching exercises may put more emphasis on one particular muscle in that muscle group, thus causing an imbalance that could lead to injury.

For example, when stretching the hamstrings (the muscles at the back of the legs) it is imperative that we keep both feet pointing up. If our feet fall to one side, this will put undue stress on one particular part of the hamstrings, which could result in a muscle imbalance.

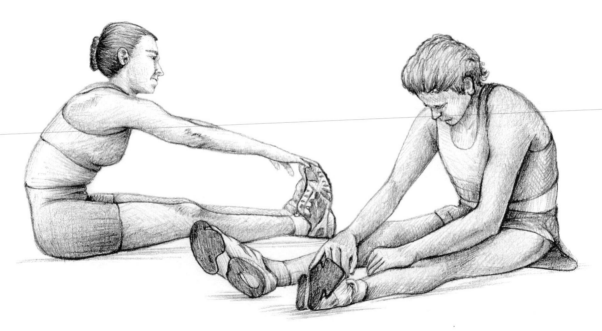

Figure 2.16: The difference between good posture and bad posture. Note the athlete on the left, feet upright and back relatively straight. The athlete on the right is at greater risk of causing a muscular imbalance that may lead to injury.

Facilities, Rules, and Protective Devices

A number of less obvious prevention techniques are often overlooked, but are equally important in helping to prevent sports injury.

Playing Areas and Facilities

These areas, designed specifically for sport and athletic activity, are often the source of unnecessary sports injuries. Broken, faulty or poorly designed equipment can lead to injury and playing surfaces that are damaged or poorly maintained put athletes at unnecessary risk.

Before participation, ensure that playing areas are free from obstructions and in good condition. Spectators should also be made aware of the importance of staying well back from playing areas.

Rules

Sporting rules are specifically designed for the protection of players and ensure a safe playing area both for participants and spectators. It is the responsibility of coaching staff, players and referees to fully understand and abide by all the rules of their particular sport.

Emphasis should also be placed on good sportsmanship, fair play and the discouragement of dangerous or violent behavior.

Protective Devices

Protective devices are designed to aid performance and reduce injuries, with all sports participation benefiting from the use of protective devices. Even the sport of running is greatly enhanced with good supportive footwear and swimmers benefit from protective eye goggles.

Other important protective devices include: mouth guards, individual player pads, helmets, shin guards, eye protection, wetsuits, goal post pads, and matting for sports that require a cushioned landing such as gymnastics.

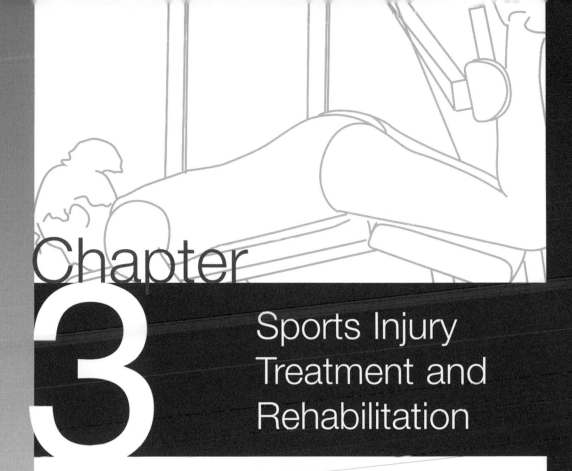

Chapter 3

Sports Injury Treatment and Rehabilitation

Introduction to Sports Injury Management

Regaining the Fitness Components

Introduction to Sports Injury Management

Sports injury management encompasses the entire process of treating a sports injury; right from the time the injury occurs, through to the time the injured player is fully recovered and 110 percent stronger and healthier than they were before the injury occurred. And no, that is not a typo. 110 percent is the goal because sports injury management should always aim to rehabilitate the injured area to the point where it is stronger after the injury, than it was before the injury.

The type of sports injuries that this management process refers to, are the soft tissue injuries, which are very common in most, if not all sports. These injuries include sprains, strains, tears and bruises that affect the muscles, tendons, ligaments and joints; or the soft tissues of the body.

Examples of common soft tissue injuries include hamstring tears, sprained ankles, pulled calf muscles, strained shoulder ligaments and corked thigh. Remember, a sprain refers to a tear or rupture of the ligaments, while a strain refers to a tear or rupture of the muscles or tendons.

The type of sports injuries that this management process *does not* refer to are injuries that affect the head, neck, face or spinal cord; injuries that involve shock, excessive bleeding, or bone fractures and breaks. The treatment of these types of injuries goes way beyond the relatively simple soft tissue injuries that are being discussed here. Although this type of serious sports injury is rare, immediate medical attention must be sought.

Soft tissue sports injury management involves four phases.

1. First aid: the first three minutes;
2. Treatment: the next three days;
3. Rehabilitation: the next three weeks;
4. Conditioning: the next three months.

1. First Aid: the First Three Minutes

The first three minutes after an injury occurs are crucial. This is the time when an initial assessment of the injury is made and appropriate steps are taken to minimize trauma and prevent further damage. This is the first priority when treating any sports injury.

Before treating any injury, whether to yourself or someone else, first STOP and take account of what has occurred. Consider things like: Is the area safe from other dangers? Is there a threat to life? Is the injury serious enough to seek emergency help? Then, using the word STOP; as an acronym:

S: (stop) Stop the injured athlete from moving. Consider stopping the sport or game if necessary.
T: (talk) Ask questions like: What happened? How did it happen? What did it feel like? Where does it hurt? Have you injured this part before?
O: (observe) Look for things like swelling, bruising, deformity and tenderness.
P: (prevent) Remember, do no further damage. Prevent further injury.

Then make an assessment of the severity of the injury.

Is it a *mild* injury? Is it a bump or bruise that does not impair the athlete's physical performance? If so, play on. Provide a few words of encouragement; monitor the injury; and apply the treatment procedures described in Chapters 4–17 just to be on the safe side.

Is it a *moderate* injury? Is it a sprain, strain or severe bruise that impairs the athlete's ability to play on? If so, get the player off the field and apply the treatment procedures described in Chapters 4–17 as soon as possible.

Is it a *severe* injury? Does the injury affect the head, neck, face or spinal cord? Does it involve shock, excessive bleeding, or bone fractures and breaks? The treatment of these types of injuries goes way beyond the relatively simple soft tissue injury treatment. Seek professional help immediately.

Once a few moments have been taken to make sure the injury is not life threatening, it is then time to start treating the injury. The sooner treatment is started, the more chance the injured athlete has of a full and complete recovery.

2. Treatment: the Next Three Days

Without a doubt, the most effective initial treatment for soft tissue injuries is the R.I.C.E.R. regimen. This involves the application of (R) rest, (I) ice, (C) compression, (E) elevation, and obtaining a (R) referral for appropriate medical treatment.

Where the R.I.C.E.R. regimen has been used immediately after the occurrence of an injury, it has been shown to significantly reduce recovery time. R.I.C.E.R. forms the first, and perhaps most important stage of injury rehabilitation, providing the early base for the complete recovery of injury.

When a soft tissue injury occurs there is a large amount of uncontrolled bleeding around the injury site. The excessive bleeding causes swelling that puts pressure on nerve endings and results in increased pain. It is exactly this process of bleeding, swelling and pain that the R.I.C.E.R. regimen will help to alleviate. This will also limit tissue damage and aid the healing process.

Rest
It is important that the injured area be kept as still as possible. If necessary support the injured area with a sling or brace. This will help to slow blood flow to the injured area and prevent any further damage.

Ice
This is by far the most important part. The application of ice will have the greatest effect on reducing bleeding, swelling and pain. Apply ice as soon as possible after the injury has occurred.

How do you apply ice? Crushed ice in a plastic bag is usually best. However, blocks of ice, commercial cold packs and bags of frozen peas will all do fine. Even cold water from a tap is better than nothing at all.

When using ice, be careful not to apply it directly to the skin. This can cause ice burns and further skin damage. Wrapping the ice in a damp towel generally provides the best protection for the skin.

How long? How often? This is the point where few people agree. The following are some figures to use as a rough guide, and then some advice from personal experience will be offered. The most common recommendation is to apply ice for 20 minutes every 2 hours for the first 48–72 hours.

These figures are a good starting point, but remember they are only a guide. A number of precautions must be taken into account, including: Some people are more sensitive to cold than others; children and elderly people have a lower tolerance to ice and cold; and people with circulatory problems are also more sensitive to ice.

The safest recommendation is that people use their own judgment when applying ice to the injured area. For some people, 20 minutes will be way too long. For others, especially well conditioned athletes, they can leave ice on for a lot longer.

The individual should make the decision as to how long the ice should stay on. People should apply ice for as long as it is comfortable. Obviously, there will be a slight discomfort from the cold, but as soon as pain or excessive discomfort is experienced, it is time to remove the ice. It is much better to apply ice for 3–5 minutes a couple of times an hour, than not at all.

Compression
Compression actually achieves two things. Firstly, it helps to reduce both the bleeding and swelling around the injured area, and secondly, it provides support for the injured area. Simply use a wide, firm, elastic, compression bandage to cover the injured part. Bandage both above and below the injured area.

Elevation

Raise the injured area above the level of the heart at all possible times. This will further help to reduce the bleeding and swelling.

Referral

If the injury is severe enough, it is important that the injured athlete consult a professional physical therapist or a qualified sports doctor for an accurate diagnosis of the injury. With an accurate diagnosis, the athlete can then move onto a specific rehabilitation program to further reduce injury time.

A Word of Warning!

Before moving on, there are a few things that must be avoided during the first 48–72 hours after an injury. Be sure to avoid any form of heat at the injury site. This includes heat lamps, heat creams, spas, jacuzzis and saunas. Avoid all movement and massage of the injured area. Also avoid excessive alcohol. All these things will increase the bleeding, swelling and pain of your injury. Avoid them at all costs.

3. Rehabilitation: the Next Three Weeks

When a muscle is torn or damaged, it would be reasonable to expect that the body would repair that damage with new muscle, or ligament, if a ligament is damaged, and so on. In reality, this does not happen. The tear, or damage, is repaired with scar tissue.

When the R.I.C.E.R. regimen is used immediately after a soft tissue injury occurs, it will limit the formation of scar tissue. However, some scar tissue will still be present.

This might not sound like a big deal, but for anyone who has ever suffered a soft tissue injury, they will know how annoying it is to keep re-injuring that same old injury, over and over again. Untreated scar tissue is the major cause of re-injury, usually months after you thought that injury had fully healed.

Scar tissue is made from a very brittle, inflexible fibrous material called collagen. This fibrous material binds itself to the damaged soft tissue fibers in an effort to draw the damaged fibers back together. What results is a bulky mass of fibrous scar tissue completely surrounding the injury site. In some cases it is even possible to see and feel this bulky mass under the skin.

When scar tissue forms around an injury site, it is never as strong as the tissue it replaces. It also has a tendency to contract and deform the surrounding tissues, so not only is the strength of the tissue diminished, but flexibility of the tissue is also compromised.

So what does this mean for the athlete? Firstly, it means a shortening of the soft tissues resulting in a loss of flexibility. Secondly, it means a weak spot has formed within the soft tissues, which could easily result in further damage or re-injury.

Lastly, the formation of scar tissue will result in a loss of strength and power. For a muscle to attain full power it must be fully stretched before contraction. Both the shortening effect and weakening of the tissues means that a full stretch and optimum contraction is not possible.

Getting Rid of the Scar Tissue

To speed up the recovery process and remove or re-align the unwanted scar tissue, two vital treatments need to be initiated.

The first is commonly used by physical therapists (or physiotherapists), and primarily involves increasing the blood supply to the injured area. The aim is to increase the amount of oxygen and nutrients to the damaged tissues. Physical therapists accomplish this aim by using a number of activities to stimulate the injured area. The most common methods used are ultrasound and heat.

Ultrasound, or *TENS* (Transcutaneous Electrical Nerve Stimulation) simply uses a light electrical pulse to stimulate the affected area. While heat, in the form of a ray lamp or hot water bottle is very effective in stimulating blood flow to the damaged tissues.

The second treatment used to remove the unwanted scar tissue is deep tissue sports massage. While ultrasound and heat will help the injured area, they will not remove the scar tissue. Only massage will do that.

Either find someone who can massage the affected area, or if the injury is accessible, massage the damaged tissues yourself. Doing this yourself has the advantage of knowing just how hard and how deep you need to massage.

To start with, the area will be quite tender. Start with a light stroke and gradually increase the pressure until deep, firm strokes can be used. Massage in the direction of the muscle fibers and concentrate the most effort at the direct point of injury. Use the thumbs to get in as deep as possible to break down the scar tissue.

Recommended for improved soft tissue recovery is a special massage ointment called *Arnica*. This ointment is extremely effective in treating soft tissue injuries, like sprains, strains and tears.

Also, be sure to drink plenty of fluid during the injury rehabilitation process. The extra fluid will help to flush a lot of the waste products from the body.

Active Rehabilitation

As part of the rehabilitation phase the injured athlete will be required to do exercises and activities that will help to speed up the recovery process. Some people refer to this phase of the recovery process as the active rehabilitation phase, because during this phase the athlete is responsible for the rehabilitation process.

The aim of this phase of the recovery will be to regain all the fitness components that were lost during the injury process. Regaining flexibility, strength, power, muscular endurance, balance, and co-ordination will be the primary focus.

Without this phase of the rehabilitation process, there is no hope of completely and permanently making a full recovery from your injury. A quote from *Sporting Injuries* by Dornan, P., and Dunn, R., will help to reinforce the value of active rehabilitation.

"The injury symptoms will permanently disappear only after the patient has undergone a very specific exercise program, deliberately designed to stretch and strengthen and regain all parameters of fitness of the damaged structure or structures. Further, it is suggested that when a specific stretching program is followed, thus more permanently reorganizing the scar fibers and allowing the circulation to become normal, the painful symptoms will disappear permanently."

The first point to make clear is how important it is to keep active. Often, the advice from doctors and similar medical personnel will be simply to rest. This can be one of the worst things an injured athlete can do. Without some form of activity the injured area will not receive the blood flow it requires for recovery. An active circulation will provide both the oxygen and nutrients needed for the injury to heal.

Any form of gentle activity not only promotes blood circulation, but also activates the lymphatic system. The lymphatic system is vital in clearing the body of toxins and waste products that accumulate in the body following a serious injury. Activity is the only way to activate the lymphatic system. Dornan and Dunn also support this approach.

"One does not need to wait for full anatomical healing before starting to retrain the muscle. The retraining can be started, gradually at first, during the healing period. This same principle applies also to ligamentous and tendon injuries."

A Word of Warning!

Never do any activity that hurts the injured area or causes pain. Of course some discomfort may be felt, but never push the injured area to the point where pain is felt. The recovery process is a long journey. Do not take a step backwards by overexerting the injured area. Be very careful with any activity. Pain is the warning sign; do not ignore it.

Regaining the Fitness Components

Now is the time to work on regaining the fitness components that were lost as a result of the injury. The main areas that need to be worked on are range of motion, flexibility, strength, and co-ordination.

Depending on the background of the athlete, and the type of sport that the athlete was engaged in, these elements should be the first priority. As the athlete starts to regain strength, flexibility and co-ordination, they can then start to work on the more specific areas of their chosen sport.

Range of Motion

Regaining a full range of motion is the first priority in this phase of the rehabilitation process. A full range of motion is extremely important, as it lays the foundation for more intense and challenging exercises later in the active rehabilitation process.

While working through the initial stages of recovery the injury will begin to heal, and the athlete can start to introduce some very gentle movement based exercises. First bending and straightening the injured area, then as this becomes more comfortable, start to incorporate rotation exercises. Turn the injured area from side to side, and rotate clockwise and anti-clockwise. Dornan and Dunn emphasize:

"It is important that gentle stretching exercises be initiated early if normal flexibility is to be regained. For example, by actively stretching bruises of the thigh to their fullest pain-free extent, adhesion formation was limited and the thigh muscles were able to return to the pre-injury range of motion."

When these range of motion exercises can be performed relatively pain free, it is time to move onto the next phase of the active rehabilitation process.

Stretch and Strengthen

At this point increased intensity is added to the range of motion exercises. The aim here is to gradually re-introduce some flexibility and strength back into the injured structures.

When attempting to increase the flexibility and strength of the injured area, be sure to approach this in a gradual, systematic way of lightly over-loading the injured area. Be careful not to over-do this type of training. Patience is required.

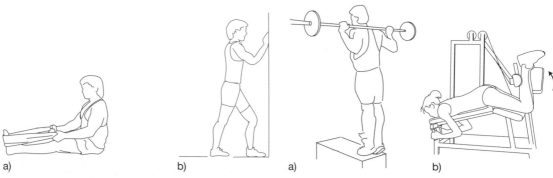

a)   b)   a)   b)

Figure 3.1: Examples of stretching;
a) thera-band stretch, b) calf stretch.

Figure 3.2: Examples of strengthening;
a) calf raise, b) leg curl.

The use of machine weights can be very effective for improving the strength of the injured area, as they provide a certain amount of stability to the joints and muscles as the athlete performs the rehabilitation exercises.

Another effective and relatively safe way to start is to begin with isometric exercises. These are exercise where the injured area does not move, yet force is applied and the muscles of the injured area are contracted.

For example: imagine sitting in a chair while facing a wall and then placing the ball of your foot against the wall. In this position you can push against the wall with your foot and at the same time keep your ankle joint from moving. The muscles contract but the ankle joint does not move. This is an isometric exercise.

It is also important at this stage to introduce some gentle stretching exercise. These will help to further increase the range of motion and prepare the injury for more strenuous activity to come.

Remember, while working on increasing the flexibility of the injured area, it is also important to increase the flexibility of the muscle groups around the injured area. In the example above, these would include the calf muscles, and the anterior muscles of the shin.

Balance and Proprioception

This phase of the rehabilitation process is often overlooked and is one of the main reasons why old injuries keep re-occurring. When a soft tissue injury occurs, there is always a certain amount of damage to the nerves around the injured area. This, of course, leads to a lack of control of the muscles and tendons, and can also affect the stability of joint structures.

Without this information the muscles, tendons and ligaments are constantly second-guessing the position of the joints and limbs around the injured area. This lack of awareness about the position of the limbs (proprioception) can lead to a re-occurrence of the same injury long after it was thought to have completely healed.

When improved flexibility and strength has returned to the injured area it is time to incorporate some balancing drills and exercises. Balancing exercises are important to help re-train the damaged nerves around the injured area. Start with simple balancing exercises like walking along a straight line, or balancing on a beam, progress to one-leg exercises like balancing on one foot, and then try the same exercises with closed eyes.

When comfortable with the above activities, try some of the more advanced exercises like wobble or rocker boards, Swiss balls, stability cushions and foam rollers.

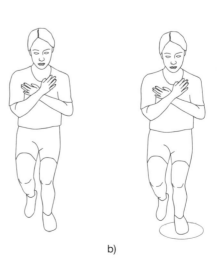

a)   b)

Figure 3.3: Examples of balance and proprioception exercises; a) keep your knee over your foot, b) add a level of difficulty by using a wobble board and closing your eyes.

Final Preparation

This last part of the rehabilitation process will aim to return the injury to a pre-injury state. By the end of this process the injured area should be as strong, if not stronger, than it was before the injury occurred.

This is the time to incorporate some dynamic or explosive exercises to really strengthen up the injured area and improve proprioception. Start by working through all the exercises done during the previous stages of recovery, but with more intensity.

For example, if you were using light isometric exercises to help strengthen the Achilles tendon and calf muscles, start to apply more force, or start to use some weighted exercises.

Next, gradually incorporate some more intense exercises. Exercises that relate specifically to the athletes chosen sport are a good place to start. Activities like skill drills and training exercises are a great way to gauge the fitness level and strength of the injured area.

To put the finishing touches on the recovery, incorporate simple plyometric drills. Plyometric exercises are explosive exercises that both lengthen and contract a muscle at the same time. These are called *eccentric muscle contractions* and involve activities like jumping, hopping, skipping and bounding.

These activities are quite intense, so remember to always start off so that you are comfortable and gradually apply more and more force. Do not get too excited and overdo it, as patience and common sense are required.

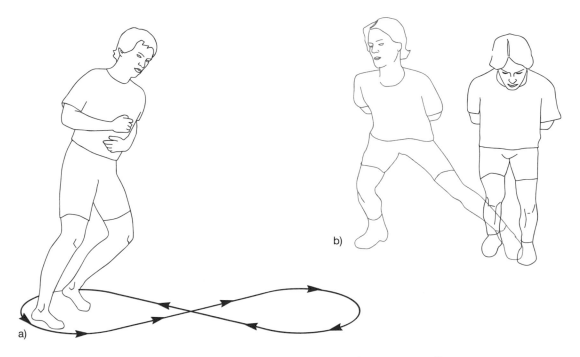

Figure 3.4: Add some more explosive exercises to aid your recovery; a) use turns specific to your sport, b) functional abductor muscle training.

4. Conditioning: the Next Three Months

Where the above treatment procedures have been diligently applied, most soft tissue injuries will have completely healed. However, even though the initial injury may have healed and the athlete is able to return to normal activities, it is important to continue further strength and conditioning exercises to prevent a repeat of the initial injury.

The goal of the next three months is to identify the underlying causes, or reasons why the injury occurred in the first place, and then once identified, employ conditioning exercises or training aids that will help to prevent a re-occurrence of the initial injury.

To accomplish this phase effectively, it is important to understand why sports injuries occur. Broadly speaking there are three main causes, or reasons why sports injuries occur. The first is *accident*, the second is *overload*, and the third is *biomechanical error*.

Accidents

Accidents include things like stepping into a pothole and spraining an ankle, tripping over and falling onto the shoulder or elbow, or being struck by sporting equipment. While there is little that can be done to prevent some accidents it is important to minimize these as much as possible. A little bit of common sense and diligently employing some of the prevention techniques in Chapter 2 will help to minimize injuries caused by accidents.

Overload

Overload is common with most sports and occurs when the structures within the body become fatigued and overworked. The structures then lose their ability to adequately perform their required task, which results in excessive strain (or overload) on other parts of the body.

For example, when the tensor fasciae latae muscle and iliotibial band, located in the thigh, become fatigued and overloaded, they lose their ability to adequately stabilize the entire leg. This in-turn places stress on the knee joint, which results in pain and damage to the structures that make up the knee joint.

Most overload symptoms can be quickly reversed with adequate rest and relaxation. However, there are a number of things that will contribute to overload and should be avoided. They include:

• Exercising on hard surfaces, like concrete;
• Exercising on uneven ground;
• Beginning an exercise program after a long lay-off period;
• Increasing exercise intensity or duration too quickly;
• Exercising in worn out or ill-fitting shoes; and,
• Excessive uphill or downhill running.

Biomechanical Error

Biomechanical errors are commonly responsible for many chronic injuries and occur when the structures within the body are not functioning as they should.

A common biomechanical error is muscle imbalance. This is where one muscle, or group of muscles, is either stronger or more flexible than its opposing muscles. This can occur on the left and right sides of the body or the front and back of the body.

For example, a right-handed baseball pitcher will commonly have overdeveloped shoulder and arm muscles on the right hand side, as compared to their left hand side. This can contribute to a pulling on the right hand side of the spine and result in chronic pain in the shoulders, neck or back.

Another common example of muscle imbalance relates to hamstring strain. This can occur when the muscles of the quadriceps (thigh muscles) are strong and powerful, yet the hamstring muscles (located in the back of the upper leg) are weak and inflexibility. Other biomechanical errors include:

- Leg length differences;
- Tight or stiff muscles;
- Foot structure problems such as flat feet; and,
- Gait or running style problems such as pronation or supination.

Once the underlying cause or reason why the injury occurred has been identified, a conditioning program or training aid can be used to correct the problem. This may involve strength or flexibility exercises in the event of weak or tight muscles. It may involve orthotics or shoe inserts in the case of pronation, supination or leg length difference. Or it may involve the modification of the athlete's current training program to prevent overload.

Chapter

4

Sports Injuries of the
Skin

001: Cuts, Abrasions, Chafing

002: Sunburn

003: Frostbite

004: Athlete's Foot (Tinea Pedis)

005: Blisters

006: Corns, Calluses, Plantar Warts (Verrucae)

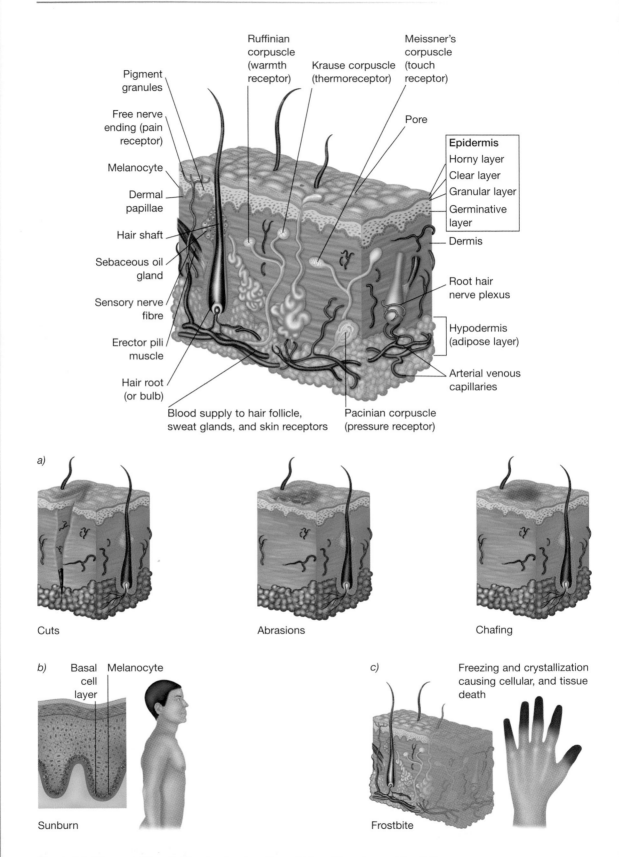

a)

Cuts

Abrasions

Chafing

b) Basal cell layer Melanocyte

Sunburn

c) Freezing and crystallization causing cellular, and tissue death

Frostbite

Figure 4.1: Cross-section of skin; a) cuts, abrasions, chafing, b) sunburn, c) frostbite.

Brief outline of injury

Skin cuts, abrasions and chafing are common afflictions among a broad variety of athletes. Such injuries involve superficial damage to the skin. The skin is broken in the case of cuts and sometimes in abrasions, while chafing is generally a surface skin phenomenon.

Anatomy and physiology

The skin is composed of two major regions. The *epidermis* consists of a number of layers of closely packed cells, containing the pigment melanin, skin, nails, sebaceous glands, and sweat glands. Its thickness depends upon its location on the body and upon where exposure to friction is greatest. The *dermis* is composed of dense irregular connective tissue, and lies between the epidermis and subcutaneous fatty tissue. It supports the epidermis structurally and nutritionally and contains collagen (the protein that helps to hold cells and tissue together). The upper part of the dermis layer has elastic fibers within connective tissue; it also has nerve-endings that are sensitive to touch. The lower portion of the dermis contains hair follicles, oil glands, ducts of sweat glands, and sensory nerve fibres.

While cuts are often caused by impact to the skin, chafing and abrasions are forms of *superficial inflammatory dermatitis*. Friction to skin leads to increased moisture and maceration. This causes a separation of keratin from the granular sublayer in the epidermis, sometimes resulting in an inflamed, oozing lesion. Generally, cuts, chafing, and abrasions to the skin do not penetrate below the epidermis, unlike *excoriation* of the skin, which affects deeper layers. Cuts and abrasions can however cause bleeding, depending on the severity of injury. Deep abrasions can also produce scarring.

Cause of injury

Friction from athletic equipment, including padding and footwear. Fall onto a hard surface. Collision with another athlete. Friction of skin against clothing, combined with sweat and other moisture.

Signs and symptoms

Redness, pain, and irritation. Itching or burning sensation. Bleeding.

Complications if left unattended

Skin injuries that are not properly treated can lead to potentially serious infections. Cuts, abrasions, and chafing combined with moisture from sweat produce an ideal medium for bacteria and viruses. Infection is further encouraged when athletic equipment obstructs the skin.

Immediate treatment

Clean affected area with soap and water, and dry thoroughly. Apply topical steroid as needed. Bandage open wounds.

Rehabilitation and prevention

Cuts often result from sudden accident such as a fall and are not preventable. Wearing properly fitting clothing and footwear, and drying areas prone to sweat with talcum or alum powders can minimize chafing and abrasions. Most chafing, cuts, and abrasions of the skin heal naturally with minimal care and attention, providing infection is avoided.

Long-term prognosis

In more severe cases, performance may be detrimentally affected. Full recovery following healing of the skin is expected in most cases.

Brief outline of injury

Ultraviolet radiation from the sun can cause damage to the skin, typically *sunburn* which can range from mild to severe. All athletes engaged in outdoor sports are vulnerable to sunburn, particularly those performing at higher altitudes where the earth's protection against ultraviolet (UV) rays is more limited. Skiers and mountaineers are hence at greater risk from the injury than athletes closer to sea level.

Anatomy and physiology

In the basal region of the skin's epidermis are dentritic cells known as *melanocytes*. Exposure to sunlight causes activity in these cells and the release of melanin, a pigment responsible for skin coloration. While gradual or less severe exposure produces tanning, excessive exposure causes damage to melanocytes, sometimes leading to a cancer of the skin known as *melanoma*.

Cause of injury

Excessive exposure to sunlight. Failure to cover exposed skin in bright sun. Failure to apply sunscreen during extended exposure.

Signs and symptoms

Redness, pain, blistering of the skin. Skin is hot to the touch.

Complications if left unattended

The most serious complication due to sunburn is melanoma, a potentially fatal cancer of the skin. Less severe complications involve damage to blood vessels, premature aging of the skin, and loss of skin elasticity.

Immediate treatment

Get out of the sun as soon as possible. Cool baths as needed and topical moisturizers, including *aloe vera*.

Rehabilitation and prevention

Sunburn is usually treated without professional attention, providing it is not severe. Moisturizer may be applied to help prevent over dryness and peeling of the skin, but the skin should not be covered with such products in the early phase of the injury while the body attempts to radiate heat. Prevent sunburn with *Slip, Slop, Slap!* Slip on a shirt, Slop on some sunscreen, and Slap on a hat.

Long-term prognosis

Most sunburn heals in a matter of days, though damaged layers may blister and peel away, with fresh skin replacing the dead layers. This new skin is particularly vulnerable to damage from the sun, and exposure should be avoided. Repeated overexposure to the sun increases the risk of skin cancer or melanoma.

Brief outline of injury

Athletes engaged in outdoor activities in cold weather are subject to frostbite, an injury caused by a freezing of body tissue, resulting in damage to the skin and subcutaneous layers. Skiers and mountaineers are particularly prone to frostbite, which tends to affect exposed skin such as nose and ears, as well as the body's extremities, but any athlete improperly protected against severe or prolonged exposure to low temperature is vulnerable.

Anatomy and physiology

Frostbite refers to the clinical condition in which water molecules within human tissue freeze and crystallize, causing cellular and tissue death. Early stages of frostbite are caused by ice formation in the extracellular tissue, causing damage to cell membranes and eventually cell and tissue death. Further freezing causes a shift in intracellular water to the extracellular space leading to dehydration and further, often irreversible damage.

Cause of injury

Prolonged exposure to the cold. Tissue getting wet and then freezing. Impeded blood flow in cold weather.

Signs and symptoms

Skin is white. Numbness or tingling, often in hands or feet. Loose and blackened skin when destroyed by frostbite.

Complications if left unattended

Severe frostbite causes permanent damage to tissue and may result in gangrene, in some cases requiring amputation.

Immediate treatment

Immerse frozen areas in warm water or apply warm compresses. Analgesics for pain.

Rehabilitation and prevention

Thawing of serious frostbite must be done carefully. Avoid rubbing the affected area. If blistering has occurred, the area should be wrapped in a sterile bandage. Do not thaw areas at risk of refreezing as more serious tissue damage may result. Frostbite is prevented by avoiding prolonged exposure to the cold or activities in extremely cold temperatures.

Long-term prognosis

Mild to moderate frostbite may leave the athlete at some increased risk for future cold sensitivity and re-injury. Severe frostbite can cause irreversible damage requiring amputation, though such injuries are usually restricted to those engaged in high altitude sports, particularly mountaineering.

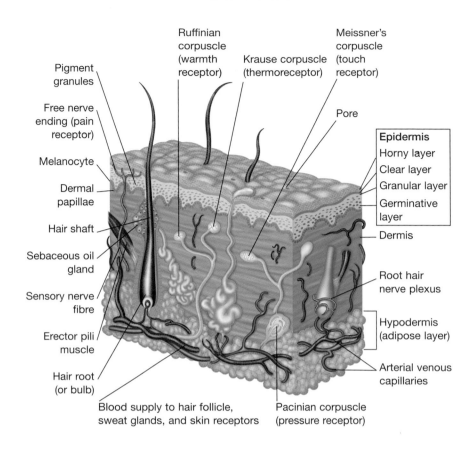

Ruffinian corpuscle (warmth receptor)

Krause corpuscle (thermoreceptor)

Meissner's corpuscle (touch receptor)

Pigment granules

Free nerve ending (pain receptor)

Pore

Melanocyte

Epidermis
Horny layer
Clear layer
Granular layer
Germinative layer

Dermal papillae

Hair shaft

Dermis

Sebaceous oil gland

Sensory nerve fibre

Root hair nerve plexus

Erector pili muscle

Hypodermis (adipose layer)

Hair root (or bulb)

Arterial venous capillaries

Blood supply to hair follicle, sweat glands, and skin receptors

Pacinian corpuscle (pressure receptor)

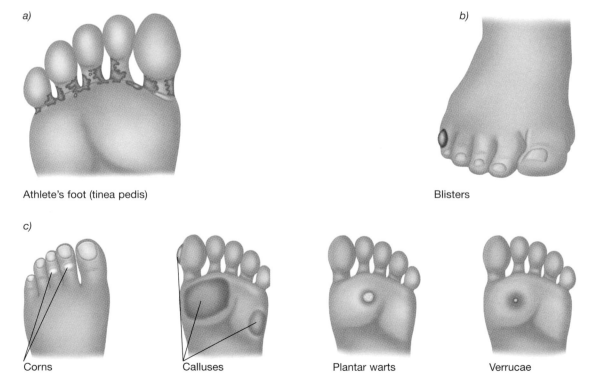

a)

Athlete's foot (tinea pedis)

b)

Blisters

c)

Corns

Calluses

Plantar warts

Verrucae

Figure 4.2: Cross-section of skin; a) athlete's foot (tinea pedis), b) blisters, c) corns, calluses, plantar warts (verrucae).

004: ATHLETE'S FOOT (TINEA PEDIS)

Brief outline of injury

Athlete's foot is caused by a fungal infection of the foot, produced by a class of parasites of the skin known as *dermatophytes*. The affliction is common among athletes and thrives in moist conditions produced by sweat. The ailment causes a red, itchy rash-like condition on the feet and may be spread to others. The most common form of the condition is known as *chronic interdigital athlete's foot*.

Anatomy and physiology

The site most commonly affected is between the spaces of the fourth and fifth toes where it causes irritation, maceration, fissures, and scaling of the outer layer of skin. Infection can spread to the dorsal and plantar surfaces of the foot and into the nails where it starts as a yellowing of the distal margin and/or along the edge of a nail. The fungi responsible are plant organisms *(tinea pedis)*, and bacteria may produce secondary infections, which worsens the symptoms.

Cause of injury

Excessive sweating. Contagious transmission. Failure to wash and properly dry the feet.

Signs and symptoms

Reddened, cracked, and peeling skin. Itching, burning, stinging sensation. Bad odour.

Complications if left unattended

Without proper care, athlete's foot can worsen, deepening the fissures in the skin, spreading across the foot surface, affecting the soles and toenails and occasionally spreading to the palms of the hands as well. The burning and itching sensation increases along with odour and the risks of spreading the ailment to others increase.

Immediate treatment

Wash and thoroughly dry the feet. Apply antifungal topical medication, e.g. *Lamicil*.

Rehabilitation and prevention

Athlete's foot is a common occurrence, affecting 70% of the population at various times. Generally, it responds well with minimal care—washing the feet often and seeing that they are thoroughly dried and whenever possible, kept dry during the day. If the nail is infected, the condition can be difficult to treat, requiring aggressive care. Chronically affected toenails may need to be removed by a podiatrist.

Long-term prognosis

Most cases of athlete's foot are resolved with proper hygiene and application of anti-fungal medication. More severe cases may require a long-term regimen of oral medication and nail removal to fully resolve the issue.

SPORTS INJURIES OF THE SKIN

Brief outline of injury

Blisters are a common injury in many sports where the skin encounters friction, either from footwear (during running events, skating, skiing, etc.) or sporting apparatus, for example, in gymnastics, baseball or racket events. Small, fluid-filled bubbles or vesicles form on the skin in response to friction. Generally, the fluid is clear but occasionally bleeding into the blister causes red or blue discolouration.

Anatomy and physiology

Blisters occur when there is a separation of the epidermis from the dermal layer of skin or a separation within the multiple layers of the epidermis itself. Serum, lymph, blood, or extracellular fluid fills the space between layers. Thin, translucent walls are formed and the area swells and may become sensitive or painful.

Cause of injury

Friction to feet from running sports. Friction to fingers and palms from golf clubs, tennis rackets, etc. Friction to hands from acrobatics and gymnastics activities.

Signs and symptoms

Raised, translucent bubbles of skin in the area of wear. Pain, stinging, and sensitivity at injury site. Leakage of fluid should blister be disturbed.

Complications if left unattended

If athletic activities are continued without attention to the blisters, they may become torn, with further irritation to the skin and resulting pain. Improperly treated blisters also run the risk of infection, as the open wound provides an ideal medium for bacteria and other germs.

Immediate treatment

Wash the blister(s) gently with soap and warm water. If needed, carefully drain fluid. Cover with sterile bandage.

Rehabilitation and prevention

Blisters generally heal with minimal care and proper attention, providing no infection has occurred. Properly fitting socks and footwear can help avoid blisters among runners. Other athletes may chalk their hands to lessen blister-causing friction, particularly in the case of gymnasts. Proper attention to athletic technique may also help minimize blisters.

Long-term prognosis

Blisters heal in a few days to a week, providing there is no serious infection. Until they have healed however, blisters can sometimes interfere with performance, due to pain and discomfort.

006: CORNS, CALLUSES, PLANTAR WARTS (VERRUCAE)

Brief outline of injury

Corns and calluses are both caused by friction and pressure – in athletes this is often due to pressure from shoes or weight bearing. Plantar warts (verrucae) result from the human papillomavirus (HPV).

Anatomy and physiology

A corn is a horny thickening of the stratum corneum of the skin of the toes, and a callus is a localized thickening of the horny layer of the epidermis due to physical trauma. Calluses often occur on weight bearing areas on the plantar surface (sole) of the foot, and may result from abnormal alignment of the metatarsal bones in the ball of the foot. Corns and calluses may have a deeper central core, or *nucleation*, which tends to be extremely tender, and are characterized by a gradual thickening and toughening of the skin, eventually leading to irritation. Warts are the result of an infection by the highly contagious human papillomavirus (HPV). Warts are epidermal lesions with a horny surface, which occur on many parts of the body, including the soles of the feet—known as *plantar's warts* or *verrucae*.

Cause of injury

Repeated friction. Weight bearing. Contagious transmission (plantar warts).

Signs and symptoms

Thickened skin where prominent bones press against the shoe (corns). Tough or thickened skin on the soles of the feet (calluses). Raised, disfigured areas of skin, on the ball, heel, and bottom of the big toe (plantar warts).

Complications if left unattended

In the case of corns and calluses, the condition may worsen, eventually causing pain requiring medical attention. Warts can spread to other body areas as well as to others.

Immediate treatment

In the case of corns and calluses, alleviate the source of pressure on the foot. In the case of verrucae, apply anti-viral medication and cover the area.

Rehabilitation and prevention

Corns and calluses are injuries directly related to pressure on the foot and are resolved by addressing the source of pressure, whether footwear, weight bearing, etc. Corns and calluses respond well to treatment, while warts or verrucae have a tendency to recur. Proper athletic footwear and attention to technique can help prevent corns and calluses while verrucae may be prevented with attention to hygiene and avoidance of environments prone to the HPV.

Long-term prognosis

Corns and calluses are usually a minor inconvenience to the athlete and clear up thoroughly once their source has been addressed. When they are a source of pain or continuing discomfort, they may be addressed through cryotherapy, excision, laser surgery or other method.

SPORTS INJURIES OF THE SKIN

Chapter

5

Sports Injuries of the
Head and Neck

Acute

007: Head Concussion, Contusion, Haemorrhage, Fracture

008: Neck Strain, Fracture, Contusion

009: Cervical Nerve Stretch Syndrome

010: Whiplash (Neck Sprain)

011: Wryneck (Acute Torticollis)

012: Slipped Disc (Acute Cervical Disc Disease)

013: Pinched Nerve (Cervical Radiculitis)

014: Spur Formation (Cervical Spondylosis)

015: Teeth

016: Eye

017: Ear

018: Nose

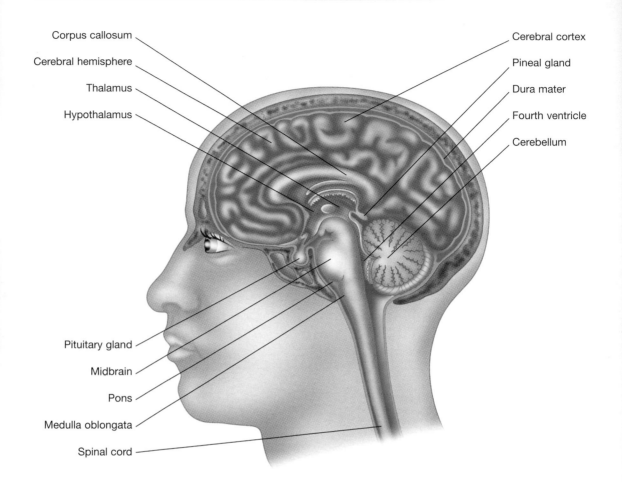

Corpus callosum

Cerebral hemisphere

Thalamus

Hypothalamus

Cerebral cortex

Pineal gland

Dura mater

Fourth ventricle

Cerebellum

Pituitary gland

Midbrain

Pons

Medulla oblongata

Spinal cord

Figure 5.1: The head, lateral view.

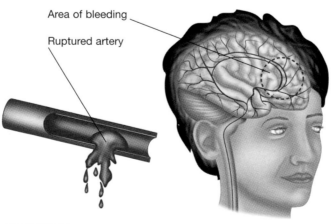

Area of bleeding

Ruptured artery

Haemorrhage

007: HEAD CONCUSSION, CONTUSION, HAEMORRHAGE, FRACTURE

Brief outline of injury

Traumas to the head are amongst the most serious injuries facing an athlete. Among these are: *concussion*, involving sudden acceleration of the head; *contusion* or bruising of the brain tissue, *haemorrhage* or bleeding inside the skull, and *fracture* or breaking of bones in the skull. Athletes engaged in contact sports such as football, rugby, lacrosse, and hockey (as well as boxers) are the most vulnerable to such injuries.

Anatomy and physiology

If the force is sufficient, bones of the skull can fracture, sometimes impinging on brain tissue. Bleeding or haemorrhage inside the skull can occur (with or without fracture). If a blood vessel lying between the skull and the brain ruptures it may form a clot or *haematoma*, which may press on the underlying brain tissue. A clot forming between the skull and the brain's protective covering or *dura mater* is known as an *epidural haematoma* while a clot below the dura is known as a *subdural haematoma*. Haemorrhage in deeper layers may cause a contusion or bruising to the brain tissue.

Cause of injury

Forceful collision with another athlete during contact sports. Serious fall with impact to the head. Trauma from blow in boxing.

Signs and symptoms

Loss of consciousness. Confusion and memory loss. Shock.

Complications if left unattended

Head injuries require immediate medical attention. Failure to seek prompt, professional care can result in permanent brain damage and, in more severe cases, fatality.

Immediate treatment

Immobilize patient, (with head and shoulders raised) in a quiet place. Stanch the flow of blood if necessary and seek immediate medical care.

Rehabilitation and prevention

Rehabilitation from head injuries varies widely depending on the nature and extent. Even mild concussions result in a post-concussion syndrome in many patients, which can persist for six months to a year. More serious injuries can cause a broad array of permanent symptoms. Helmets or other appropriate headgear in sports where the skull is vulnerable help prevent such injuries.

Long-term prognosis

Prognosis for a head injury may not be fully known for months or, in some cases, years. In the case of a mild injury, the prognosis is generally good, though symptoms including headache, dizziness, and amnesia may persist. Blood clots, haemorrhaging, and fractures of the skull often require surgery.

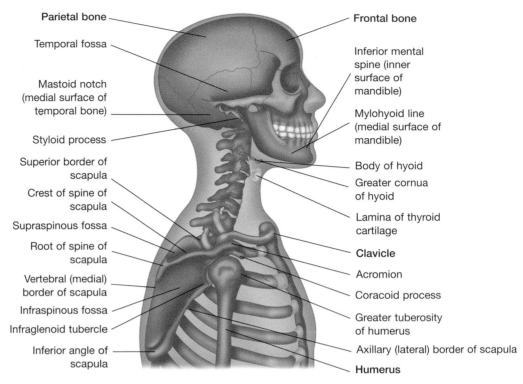

Parietal bone

Temporal fossa

Mastoid notch (medial surface of temporal bone)

Styloid process

Superior border of scapula

Crest of spine of scapula

Supraspinous fossa

Root of spine of scapula

Vertebral (medial) border of scapula

Infraspinous fossa

Infraglenoid tubercle

Inferior angle of scapula

Frontal bone

Inferior mental spine (inner surface of mandible)

Mylohyoid line (medial surface of mandible)

Body of hyoid

Greater cornua of hyoid

Lamina of thyroid cartilage

Clavicle

Acromion

Coracoid process

Greater tuberosity of humerus

Axillary (lateral) border of scapula

Humerus

Figure 5.2: Head and neck, lateral view.

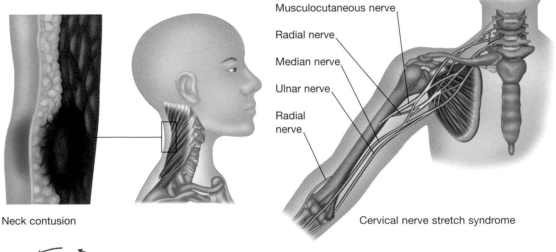

Musculocutaneous nerve

Radial nerve

Median nerve

Ulnar nerve

Radial nerve

Cervical nerve stretch syndrome

Neck contusion

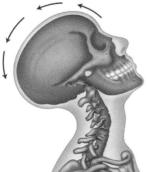

Whiplash (neck sprain)

008: NECK STRAIN, FRACTURE, CONTUSION

Brief outline of injury

Injuries to the neck can be serious, particularly in the case of broken or fractured vertebrae. Neck strains are less serious and far more common and involve injury to the muscles or tendons of the neck. Contusions are bruises to the skin and underlying tissue of the neck, usually the result of a direct blow.

Anatomy and physiology

The cervical spine is made up of seven vertebrae, which begin at the base of the skull (C1) and curve downward slightly as they reach the chest region and connect with the thoracic vertebrae (C7). Muscles running from the rib cage and collarbone to the cervical vertebrae, jaw, and skull appear on the front or anterior cervical area. The posterior cervical muscles cover the bones along the back of the spine and make up the bulk of the tissues on the back of the neck.

Cause of injury

Sudden twisting of the neck. Serious fall. Direct blow to the neck, in the case of contusion.

Signs and symptoms

Head, neck, and shoulder pain. Crackling sensation in the neck. Loss of neck strength and mobility.

Complications if left unattended

Injuries to the neck are potentially serious and deserve prompt medical attention. Long-term paralysis, loss of motion and coordination, calcification and osteoporosis are possible side-effects. In the case of fracture, the injury can lead to paraplegia and is also sometimes fatal.

Immediate treatment

Immobilization to protect the spinal cord. Analgesics for pain.

Rehabilitation and prevention

For neck strains, immobilization for a period of weeks with a brace may be recommended. In cases of fracture, the broken vertebrae may be surgically pinned together with screws and the patient may be placed in a neck cast. Physical therapy following healing will attempt to re-establish range of motion, flexibility, and strength. Helmets or other athletic headgear as well as attention to proper technique can help prevent some neck injuries.

Long-term prognosis

Outcomes for neck injury vary widely depending on the nature and severity. In cases of fracture, the prognosis is generally worse with injuries occurring higher up the cervical spine.

Neck strains and contusions are far less serious and their outcome—given proper treatment and rehabilitation—is usually good. Severe strains in which the muscle-tendon-bone attachment is ruptured may require surgical repair.

009: CERVICAL NERVE STRETCH SYNDROME

Brief outline of injury

Cervical nerve stretch syndrome, also sometimes referred to as *burner syndrome*, results from the stretching (or compression) of the *brachial plexus*; a complex of nerves in the lower neck and shoulder area. The injury is common in contact sports including hockey, football, wrestling, and rugby. Sports injuries to the brachial plexus are characterized by a burning sensation that radiates down an upper extremity. Symptoms may last anywhere from two minutes to two weeks.

Anatomy and physiology

The brachial plexus are nerves originating in the brain. They exit the cervical vertebrae, extending to peripheral structures including muscles and organs, (to which they transmit motor and sensory nerve impulses). A series of cervical nerve roots within the brachial plexus send fibers to the shoulder and trapezius muscle, the deltoid muscle and distal radius, the elbow, and the fingers.

Cause of injury

Blow to the head or shoulder, especially in a football tackle. Ear to shoulder bending with rotation (compression of cervical nerves). Hyperextension of the neck.

Signs and symptoms

Severe, burning pain, radiating from the neck to the arm and/or fingers. *Parasthesia* or numbness, tingling, pricking, burning, or creeping sensation of the skin. Muscle weakness.

Complications if left unattended

Burning and stinging symptoms will persist and often worsen. Further damage to peripheral nerves can result should the injury be ignored. Symptoms may also indicate spinal cord injury, with potentially serious complications.

Immediate treatment

Ice and immobilize the neck region. Anti-inflammatory medication and analgesics for pain.

Rehabilitation and prevention

Rehabilitation for cervical nerve stretch syndrome usually entails physical therapy. Following a healing phase, such therapy seeks to improve cervical range of motion and to strengthen cervical muscles, with particular attention to the muscles supporting the injured brachial plexus nerve. Proper protective gear, appropriate technique and upper-extremity strength training can help prevent the injury.

Long-term prognosis

Prognosis for the injury is generally good, though some athletes develop a chronic form of the condition and a high rate of recurrence has also been noted. In rare cases, nerve injury requires microsurgery to repair nerve damage.

Rehabilitation exercises

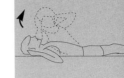
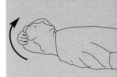
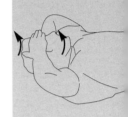
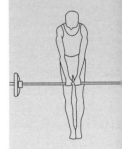
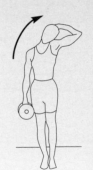

010: WHIPLASH (NECK SPRAIN)

Rehabilitation exercises

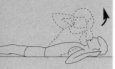

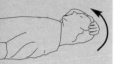

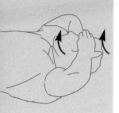

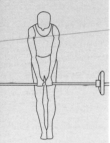

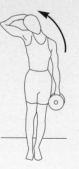

Brief outline of injury

Whiplash injury occurs when there is sudden flexion and/or extension of the neck, usually when the athlete is struck from behind during contact sports and the head is rapidly thrown both forward and backward. Soft tissues of the neck including intervertebral joints, discs, ligaments, cervical muscles, and nerve roots may be injured, producing neck pain, stiffness, and loss of mobility.

Anatomy and physiology

The hips, back, and trunk are the first body segments and joints to experience movement during a whiplash. Forward motion in these structures is accompanied by upward motion, which acts to compress the cervical spine. This combined motion causes the head to revolve backward into extension, producing tension where the lower cervical segment extends and the upper cervical segment flexes. With this rotation of the cervical vertebrae, the anterior structures are separated and posterior components including facet joints are severely compressed.

Cause of injury

Tackle from behind, e.g. football. Sharp collision with another athlete or piece of equipment. Blow to the head, e.g. boxing.

Signs and symptoms

Pain and stiffness in the neck, shoulder or between the shoulder-blades. Ringing in the ears or blurred vision. Irritability and fatigue.

Complications if left unattended

Left untreated, whiplash injury can produce chronic symptoms of pain, inflexibility and loss of movement, along with the continuation or worsening of associated symptoms of fatigue, sleep loss, memory and concentration loss, and depression. Symptoms may also suggest more serious injury to the spinal vertebrae with potentially serious consequences.

Immediate treatment

R.I.C.E.R. procedure. Immobilization with a cervical collar.

Rehabilitation and prevention

The neck will usually be immobilized with some form of brace, though early movement is usually encouraged to prevent stiffening. Low impact strength and flexibility training and rehabilitation should follow complete healing of the tendons, discs, and ligaments. Risk of whiplash may be minimized with protective gear as well as a thorough warm-up routine, though prevention in rough contact sports may not be guaranteed.

Long-term prognosis

The long-term prognosis for most whiplash injuries is good, given adequate care, though symptoms may persist and the neck may be prone to re-injury.

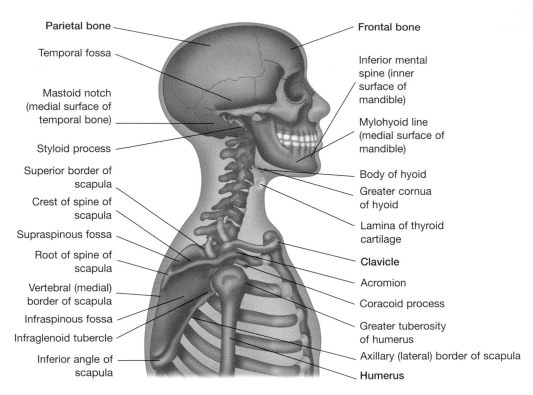

Parietal bone

Temporal fossa

Mastoid notch
(medial surface of
temporal bone)

Styloid process

Superior border of
scapula

Crest of spine of
scapula

Supraspinous fossa

Root of spine of
scapula

Vertebral (medial)
border of scapula

Infraspinous fossa

Infraglenoid tubercle

Inferior angle of
scapula

Frontal bone

Inferior mental
spine (inner
surface of
mandible)

Mylohyoid line
(medial surface of
mandible)

Body of hyoid

Greater cornua
of hyoid

Lamina of thyroid
cartilage

Clavicle

Acromion

Coracoid process

Greater tuberosity
of humerus

Axillary (lateral) border of scapula

Humerus

Figure 5.3: Skull to humerus, lateral view.

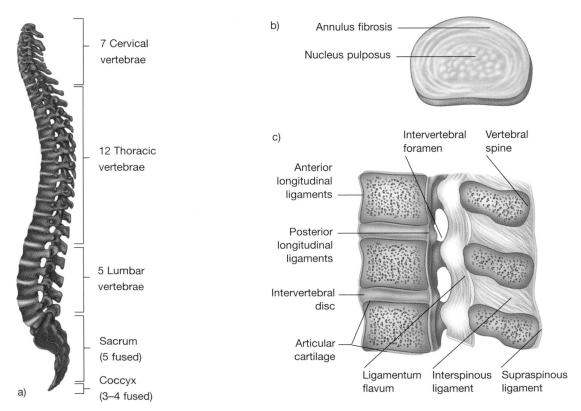

7 Cervical vertebrae

12 Thoracic vertebrae

5 Lumbar vertebrae

Sacrum (5 fused)

Coccyx (3–4 fused)

b) Annulus fibrosis

Nucleus pulposus

c)

Intervertebral foramen

Vertebral spine

Anterior longitudinal ligaments

Posterior longitudinal ligaments

Intervertebral disc

Articular cartilage

Ligamentum flavum

Interspinous ligament

Supraspinous ligament

a)

Figure 5.4; a) The vertebral column, lateral view, b) transverse section of a lumbar intervertebral disc,
c) sagittal section through 2nd to 4th lumbar vertebrae.

011: WRYNECK (ACUTE TORTICOLLIS)

Rehabilitation exercises

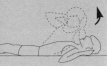

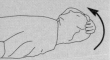

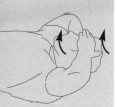

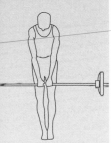

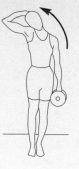

Brief outline of injury

Wryneck or *acute torticollis* is a painful neck injury that usually follows a sudden rotational movement of the head. Nerves in the neck are compressed, resulting in muscle spasms, accompanying pain, and loss of movement. Many sports can cause the injury, though it can often arise spontaneously in the morning when waking up. In the first case, the injury is usually joint-related; whilst *slow-onset torticollis* (as after sleep) is often disc-related.

Anatomy and physiology

Whilst irritation of the discs of the cervical spine, or disc prolapse (rupturing), can lead to the condition, a sudden injury, as during sports activity, is usually the result of compression of the nerves in the neck or a sprain in one of the joint facets. Typically, the neck is frozen in one position, often rotated to one side and bent forward by the contraction of the cervical muscles.

Cause of injury

Sudden rotation of the head in contact sports. A fall that causes a sudden torsion in the neck. Direct blow to the head, causing sudden twisting.

Signs and symptoms

Pain and stiffness. Loss of motion. Neck may be stuck or frozen in one position.

Complications If left unattended

Wryneck can worsen, in some cases becoming chronic if ignored. The condition may indicate damage to the cervical vertebrae, cervical discs or associated nerves and joints, requiring medical attention.

Immediate treatment

Immobilization of the injured neck with a brace or supportive cervical collar. Anti-inflammatory medication and ice to reduce swelling.

Rehabilitation and prevention

It is critical to determine the cause of the injury and rule out serious underlying conditions requiring surgery or major medical intervention. Following this, a physical therapist may use an infrared heat lamp as well as massage of the cervical vertebrae in order to restore range of motion in the injured neck. Protective headgear, upper body and neck strengthening and attention to proper athletic technique may help reduce the likelihood of this injury.

Long-term prognosis

Wryneck usually resolves in a week or less, though the painful spasms can be temporarily debilitating. While a chronic form of the condition exists, for most, full recovery can be expected, barring more serious underlying conditions.

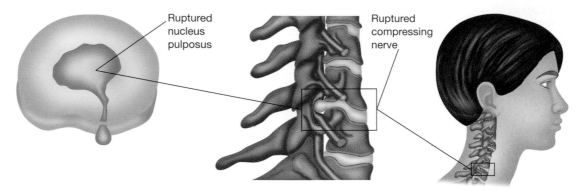

Ruptured
nucleus
pulposus

Ruptured
compressing
nerve

Slipped disc (acute cervical disc disease)

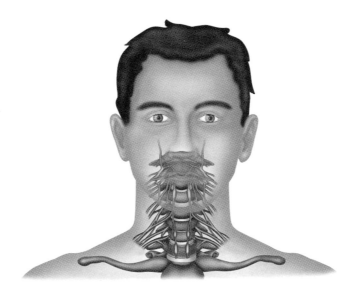

Pinched nerve (cervical radiculitis)

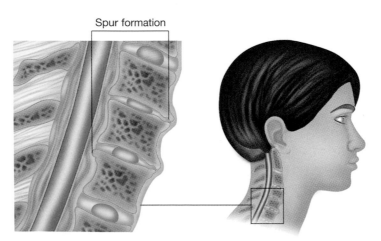

Spur formation

Spur formation (cervical spondylosis)

012: SLIPPED DISC (ACUTE CERVICAL DISC DISEASE)

Rehabilitation exercises

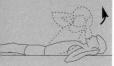

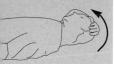

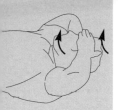

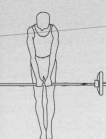

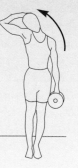

Brief outline of injury

Cervical discs are shock-absorbing pads of tissue cushioning bones of the cervical spine. A variety of injuries to these discs can cause pain and hamper movement and flexibility of the neck. Slipped discs occur when the gel-like substance leaks from the disc's interior, following a split or rupture to the disc. This substance can then exert pressure on the spinal cord or nerves of the cervical spine.

Anatomy and physiology

The intervertebral discs absorb shock, facilitate movement, and provide support for the spinal column. Such discs consist of a center region or *nucleus pulposus* and a surrounding *annulus fibrosis* separating each segmental vertebra between the C2–T1 (see page 70). (Only ligaments and joint capsules exist between C1 and C2). Disc *degeneration* and/or *herniation* (disc rupture) can cause injury to the spinal cord or nerve roots.

Cause of injury

Disc degeneration and loss of elasticity. Repetitive stress, particularly from excessive or improper weight lifting. Sudden, forceful trauma to the cervical vertebrae.

Signs and symptoms

Tingling and weakness. Numbness or pain in the neck, shoulder, arm, or hand. Motor and sensory dysfunction in the affected cervical area.

Complications if left unattended

Herniated or slipped discs can impinge on the spinal cord, an extremely delicate structure. Even minor damage to the spinal cord can be serious and is generally not reparable. Ignoring cervical disc injuries can lead to further degeneration and associated pain and mobility loss.

Immediate treatment

Discontinue activity causing stress to cervical vertebrae and discs. Rest, ice and use of anti-inflammatory medication.

Rehabilitation and prevention

For most slipped disc injuries, a conservative course of treatment is undertaken. The neck may be immobilized for a period in a cervical collar during healing. Physical therapy includes stretching, strengthening and proprioceptive exercises and sometimes, efforts to adjust posture. Upper body exercise may help prevent disc hardening and degeneration, while strengthening supporting muscles will lower the risk of rupture.

Long-term prognosis

The majority of slipped or herniated disc injuries improve without recourse to surgery. Most athletes can expect a full return to normal performance following rest and rehabilitation, though symptoms of the injury occasionally recur and degenerated discs are prone to re-rupturing.

013: PINCHED NERVE (CERVICAL RADICULITIS)

Brief outline of injury

Nerves controlling the shoulder, arm and hand originate within the spinal cord in the neck. Inflammation or compression of one of these structures is known as a pinched nerve or *cervical radiculitis*, and results in pain, weakness, and loss of movement. Herniation of the cervical discs—often caused by repetitive stress—can impinge on the cervical nerves, also causing the injury.

Anatomy and physiology

Cervical radiculitis occurs when a disc from one of the seven cervical vertebrae making up the upper spine presses against the spinal nerves connecting to the spinal cord. Such nerves branch to numerous areas of the body, and symptoms may radiate from the source along the nerve to areas where the nerve travels. Depending on the affected disc impinging on the cervical nerve, pain may occur in the arm, chest, neck, or shoulders.

Cause of injury

Herniated disc pressing on a nerve. Irritation of the nerve due to repetitive stress. Bone spurs or degenerating vertebrae impinging on a nerve.

Signs and symptoms

Pain, weakness, and loss of movement in the neck. Numb fingers. Weak muscles in the arms and chest.

Complications if left unattended

Inflammation and pain associated with pinched nerves may continue or worsen, should the source of the injury not be addressed. The nerve may become permanently damaged through continued pressure and stress, and the condition may point to other (potentially serious) underlying injuries to the vertebrae or spinal cord.

Immediate treatment

Cease activity stressful to the cervical spine. Rest, ice, analgesics, and anti-inflammatory medication.

Rehabilitation and prevention

Given proper treatment, the prognosis for cervical radiculitis is generally good. Mild cases usually respond to physical therapy in conjunction with medications such as NSAIDs or steroids. Following healing, a program of physical therapy and flexibility/strengthening exercises can help restore the athlete's former condition. Attention to proper technique, particularly during weight training/weight lifting can help prevent pinched nerve injury.

Long-term prognosis

Most cervical pinched nerve injuries resolve themselves without serious medical intervention. More serious or prolonged cases may require surgery to relieve compression of the nerve root.

**Rehabilitation
exercises**

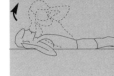
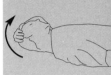
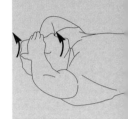
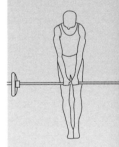
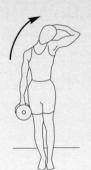

014: SPUR FORMATION (CERVICAL SPONDYLOSIS)

Rehabilitation exercises

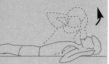
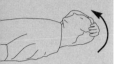
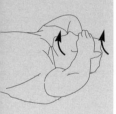
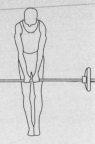
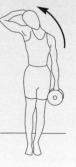

Brief outline of injury

Cervical spondylosis is a chronic degeneration of the vertebrae of the neck (cervical spine) and the intervertebral cushions or discs. Bone spurs, or *osteophytes*, are bony projections that form along joints and are often associated with arthritis. Such spurs themselves can rub against nearby nerves or occasionally on the spinal cord, causing pain and limitations in joint motion. The degeneration results from wear on the bones of the cervical spine over time.

Anatomy and physiology

Aging and repetitive stress can cause discs of the spine to become drier and less elastic. Such degeneration may cause discs to bulge or in some cases, rupture. When the surrounding ligaments become less flexible, the vertebrae develop bone spurs—new areas of bone growth along the margins of existing bones.

Cause of injury

Repetitive wear on cervical vertebrae. Excessive or improper weight lifting. Bulging or herniated cervical disc.

Signs and symptoms

Neck pain radiating to shoulders and arms. Loss of balance. Headaches radiating to the back of the head.

Complications if left unattended

Cervical spondylosis is a common cause of spinal cord dysfunction in older adults. If the condition isn't treated, the injury may progress and become permanent. Bone spurs or herniated discs can impinge and put pressure on the roots of one or more nerves of the spinal cord in the neck, producing tingling, burning, weakness or numbness in the arms or hands. Displaced spurs can also float in the system, periodically interfering with joints.

Immediate treatment

Neck brace or cervical collar to help limit neck motion. NSAIDs.

Rehabilitation and prevention

Less serious cases of cervical spondylosis respond to exercises prescribed by a physical therapist, aimed at strengthening and stretching neck muscles. Low-impact aerobic exercises including walking or swimming may also help. While age-related spondylosis may be difficult to prevent, minimizing high impact activity, engaging in upper body training and attention to posture may help avoid the injury.

Long-term prognosis

Mild cases of cervical spondylosis respond well after immobilization of the injury and appropriate physical therapy. More serious cases may require injections of corticosteroids between the vertebral facet joints or in some cases, surgery to remove bone spurs, particularly if they have broken off from larger sections of bone to become loose bodies.

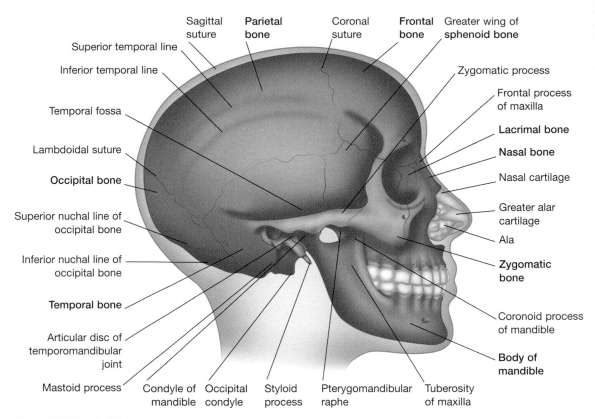

Sagittal suture

Superior temporal line

Inferior temporal line

Temporal fossa

Lambdoidal suture

Occipital bone

Superior nuchal line of occipital bone

Inferior nuchal line of occipital bone

Temporal bone

Articular disc of temporomandibular joint

Mastoid process

Condyle of mandible

Occipital condyle

Styloid process

Pterygomandibular raphe

Tuberosity of maxilla

Parietal bone

Coronal suture

Frontal bone

Greater wing of sphenoid bone

Zygomatic process

Frontal process of maxilla

Lacrimal bone

Nasal bone

Nasal cartilage

Greater alar cartilage

Ala

Zygomatic bone

Coronoid process of mandible

Body of mandible

Figure 5.5: The skull, lateral view.

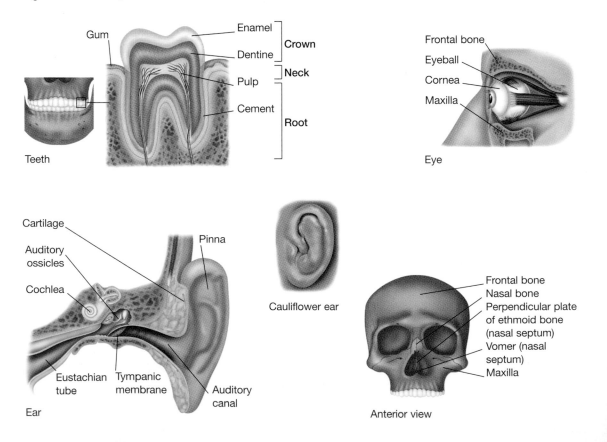

Gum

Enamel

Dentine

Pulp

Cement

Crown

Neck

Root

Teeth

Frontal bone

Eyeball

Cornea

Maxilla

Eye

Cartilage

Auditory ossicles

Cochlea

Pinna

Eustachian tube

Tympanic membrane

Auditory canal

Ear

Cauliflower ear

Frontal bone

Nasal bone

Perpendicular plate of ethmoid bone (nasal septum)

Vomer (nasal septum)

Maxilla

Anterior view

Brief outline of injury

Injury to the teeth is a particular risk for athletes involved in sports where a projectile such as a ball or puck can strike the player's face. Such sports include hockey, lacrosse, and football. The most common injuries of this sort are a *fractured, displaced* or *avulsed* (knocked out) tooth. Injuries to the teeth often accompany other head and neck injuries, including fractured facial bones, concussions, abrasions, bruises, soft tissue lacerations with bleeding, and jaw-joint problems.

Anatomy and physiology

Teeth are any of the hard, calcified structures set in the alveolar processes of the mandible and maxilla. Each tooth consists of the crown, the neck, and the root. The solid part includes *dentin*, which forms most of the tooth, the *enamel*, which covers the crown, and *cementum*, covering the root. In the center is the *soft pulp*. Teeth can be chipped or in some cases, knocked out altogether, given sufficient force from a bat or ball, etc. The avulsed tooth runs the risk of being rejected by the body as a foreign object and should therefore be cleaned and replaced firmly in its socket as soon after the injury as possible.

Cause of injury

Teeth struck with a ball, puck or other projectile. Direct blow in boxing. Teeth struck by equipment including bats, sticks, racquets, etc.

Signs and symptoms

Mouth pain. Loose teeth. Bleeding from the mouth.

Complications if left unattended

Injury to the teeth should receive prompt medical attention, particularly if a tooth is lost during sports, as host rejection of the tooth will prevent its later replacement. Swallowing a tooth after injury is a danger as is infection in the mouth if the injury is not properly cleaned and attended to.

Immediate treatment

If the tooth has been knocked out, wash in saline and replace firmly in the socket. Rinse mouth and use analgesics and ice for pain relief.

Rehabilitation and prevention

Rehabilitation from injury to the teeth is dependent on the nature and severity. Chipped or fractured teeth can be repaired and bonded by a dentist and lost teeth replaced. The athlete should refrain from activities that put the teeth at risk until thorough healing has been accomplished. Use of a mouth guard, particularly a custom-fitted one, helps protect the teeth during high risk and contact sports.

Long-term prognosis

Most injuries to the teeth, while painful, do not threaten an athlete's career or future performance, particularly provided they are given proper medical and dental attention. A knocked out tooth has a good prognosis for replanting, providing this is done within the first thirty minutes of the injury. After more than two hours, the prognosis is poor for tooth replacement, due to rejection of the tooth and re-absorption of the root.

Brief outline of injury

Injuries to the eye are always potentially serious. Many sports entail risk to the eyes, particularly those involving a ball, puck, stick, bat or racquet or other apparatus, such as a fencing foil. Basketball and baseball cause the most eye injuries, while sports carrying a low risk of injury to the eye include track and field, swimming, gymnastics, and cycling. Exposure of the eyes to excess ultraviolet (UV) radiation can also cause damage, necessitating protection of the eyes in sports like skiing and mountaineering.

Anatomy and physiology

The eyes, among the body's most delicate structures, are protected by design from injury. The eyeball is a large sphere, and is recessed in a socket surrounded by a strong, bony ridge, with the segment of a smaller sphere, the *cornea*, in front. The eyelids can close quickly, protecting the eyeball from foreign objects. Furthermore, the eye is designed to withstand some impact without serious damage. Nevertheless, even minor eye injuries can impair vision and complications can result in visual deficit or loss.

Cause of injury

Blunt trauma to the eye from equipment or direct contact, e.g. wrestling. Penetrating injury to the eye. Radiation damage due to sun overexposure.

Signs and symptoms

Blurred or absent vision. Pain or sensitivity in the eye. Obvious trauma, including bruising or bleeding.

Complications if left unattended

Eye injuries require immediate medical attention. Failure to seek medical treatment can result in visual impairment, deficit or permanent loss, particularly if ocular haemorrhaging results following the injury.

Immediate treatment

Cold compress. Avoid pressure on the eye. Seek immediate emergency medical care.

Rehabilitation and prevention

Rehabilitation for an eye injury varies broadly depending on the nature and severity. Minor injuries are generally self-healing, while serious injuries may require ophthalmic surgery and considerable rehabilitation. Eye protection including safety goggles, helmets with eye shields, or other eye protection for sports such as baseball, wrestling, football, soccer, hockey, lacrosse, paintball, basketball, and racquet sports including tennis, should always be worn to prevent such injuries.

Long-term prognosis

Prognosis for eye injuries varies according to the nature and severity. Minor injuries that do not damage underlying structures in the eye generally heal, given proper attention. More serious injuries, particularly penetrating injuries, run the risk of producing permanent visual loss, and must be treated aggressively as soon after the injury as possible.

Brief outline of injury

Injuries to the ear can occur when the ear is exposed to direct trauma (from a ball, puck, stick or other object) or through a blow in boxing or as a result of infection to the ear, as in the case of *swimmer's ear*. Cuts and lacerations to the ear are possible in a variety of athletic events, particularly contact sports, as are bruises and swelling. The eardrum can be ruptured, though this injury in sports is uncommon.

Anatomy and physiology

The ear is the human organ responsible for hearing, also playing a critical role in balance (equilibrium). Injury to the ear can affect either or both of these qualities. The outer ear consists of the outer cartilage (*pinna*) and the *auditory canal*. The middle ear consists of the *tympanic membrane* (or eardrum), the *auditory ossicles* or bones of the ear, the *middle ear cavity* and the *Eustachian tube*. Sports injuries tend to involve the outer or middle ear, rather than the inner ear, where the cochlea and other structures reside. For example, *cauliflower ear* is caused by repeated blunt trauma, where a haematoma forms between the perichondrium and the cartilage of the ear.

Cause of injury

Blow to the ear from a ball or other projectile. Sudden pressure change resulting in a ruptured eardrum. Trauma from boxing blow.

Signs and symptoms

Bleeding, swelling. Hearing loss or ringing in the ears. Dizziness and loss of balance.

Complications if left unattended

Ear injuries have potentially serious consequences for long-term hearing and should not be ignored. Ruptured eardrums can also lead to infection, with potentially serious implications.

Immediate treatment

Apply direct pressure should bleeding occur. Sterile cotton in the outer ear to keep the inside of the ear clean.

Rehabilitation and prevention

Cuts and abrasions to the ear as well as cauliflower ear usually heal with minimal medical attention. A ruptured eardrum requires particular care to avoid infection. Ear infections common to swimmers may require antibiotics and usually a period out of the water until the condition is fully resolved. Use of helmets or other headgear in contact sports helps to prevent direct trauma to the ear.

Long-term prognosis

Most athletes experiencing injury to the ear can expect a full recovery, though in the case of a ruptured eardrum, partial or in some cases, total hearing loss may result. Prompt medical attention is critical for such injuries.

SPORTS INJURIES OF THE HEAD AND NECK

Brief outline of injury

Nasal injuries are among the more common in sports, partly due to the protrusion of the nasal bones from the face. Injuries to the nose are generally due to direct blows in contact sports, from baseballs, basketballs and other athletic equipment or from a fall on the face. In addition to surface cuts, bruising and lacerations to the skin, the nasal bones may be fractured. Blood clotting beneath the mucus membranes of the septum is also possible and is known as a *septal haematoma*.

Anatomy and physiology

The nose is comprised of bone and cartilage. The *nasal septum* is often injured in sports. It consists of the *vomer*, a perpendicular plate of the *ethmoid*, and the *quadrangular cartilage*. A pair of protrusions from the frontal bones and the ascending processes of the maxilla complete the bony component, while the upper lateral and lower lateral cartilages, as well as the *cartilaginous septum*, make up the non-bony portion. *Epistaxis*, or a nosebleed, occurs when superficial blood vessels on the anterior septum are lacerated.

Cause of injury

Blow to the nose from a baseball, basketball or similar object. Blow to the nose from boxing, or during contact sports. Fall on the face.

Signs and symptoms

Nasal deformity. Bleeding, pain, or difficulty breathing. Swelling and skin laceration.

Complications if left unattended

Injuries to the nose are potentially dangerous and require prompt medical attention. Collections of clotted blood can accumulate in the *subperichondrial space*, forming a septal haematoma. Resulting pressure on the underlying cartilage can produce irreversible necrosis of the septum. There is also significant risk for infection. If the injury involves damage to the cribriform plate, the patient can lose cerebrospinal fluid, placing him at risk from meningitis or other serious complications.

Immediate treatment

Apply ice to the nose and elevate the head. Use nasal decongestants to reduce swelling and mucosal congestion.

Rehabilitation and prevention

Most injuries to the nose undergo thorough healing, though the athlete should avoid contact or other high-risk sports during this phase. Fractures need to be reset, but do not in most cases require surgery. Helmets with adequate face protection should be used where the nose is at risk, to help prevent such injuries.

Long-term prognosis

Less serious nasal injuries usually allow the athlete to return to non-contact sports within two weeks. Full healing of fractures usually occurs in three weeks, generally, without lasting cosmetic or functional deformity.

Chapter

6

Sports Injuries of the
Hands and
Fingers

Acute

019: Metacarpal Fractures

020: Thumb Sprain (Ulnar Collateral Ligament)

021: Mallet Finger (Long Extensor Tendon)

022: Finger Sprain

023: Finger Dislocation

Chronic

024: Hand / Finger Tendinitis

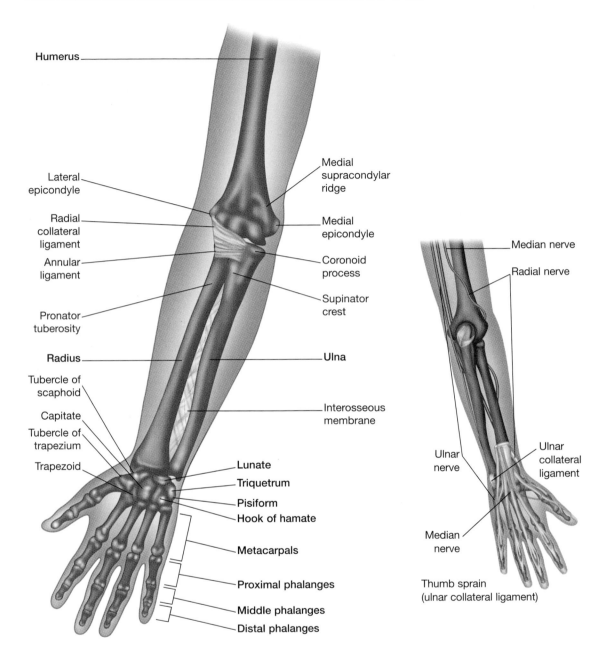

Humerus

Medial
supracondylar
ridge

Lateral
epicondyle

Medial
epicondyle

Radial
collateral
ligament

Annular
ligament

Coronoid
process

Supinator
crest

Pronator
tuberosity

Radius

Ulna

Tubercle of
scaphoid

Interosseous
membrane

Capitate

Tubercle of
trapezium

Trapezoid

Lunate

Triquetrum

Pisiform

Hook of hamate

Metacarpals

Proximal phalanges

Middle phalanges

Distal phalanges

Median nerve

Radial nerve

Ulnar
nerve

Ulnar
collateral
ligament

Median
nerve

Thumb sprain
(ulnar collateral ligament)

Figure 6.1: The bones of the right forearm and hand, anterior view.

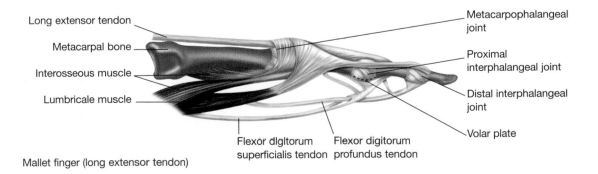

Long extensor tendon

Metacarpal bone

Interosseous muscle

Lumbricale muscle

Metacarpophalangeal
joint

Proximal
interphalangeal joint

Distal interphalangeal
joint

Volar plate

Flexor digitorum
superficialis tendon

Flexor digitorum
profundus tendon

Mallet finger (long extensor tendon)

019: METACARPAL FRACTURES

Rehabilitation exercises

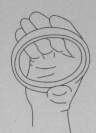

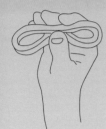

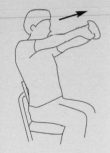

Brief outline of injury

Breaks or fractures in one or more of the metacarpal bones may result from a variety of events. They are common in football and basketball players. Metacarpals are vulnerable to direct force and can be fractured when a closed fist strikes another person or hard object, such injuries being referred to as *boxer's fracture*. Metacarpal bones can fracture either at the base, shaft or neck. The most common fracture is of the neck of the fifth metacarpal.

Anatomy and physiology

The five metacarpal bones run between the wrist and the knuckles (which are the heads of the metacarpals). Each metacarpal bone comprises a *base, shaft, neck* and *head*, (from proximal to distal end). The first metacarpal bone is the shortest and most agile, and connects with the *trapezium* at the proximal end of the thumb. The other four metacarpals of the hand connect to the *trapezoid, capitate* and *hamate*, and lateral-medial surfaces of metacarpal bones. Each finger has three phalanges, whereas the thumb only has two, making a total of fourteen phalanges. These connect with the heads of the metacarpals, forming the knuckles when the fist is closed.

Cause of injury

A direct blow to the hand. Falling directly onto the hand. Longitudinal force transmitted through a closed fist when punching.

Signs and symptoms

Local pain and swelling. Bruising and deformity of the broken bone or knuckle. Loss of hand movement and function in the affected region.

Complications if left unattended

Use of a hand not properly immobilized following metacarpal fracture may lead to lasting deformity and reduced function as well as possible damage to surrounding nerves, muscles, tendons, blood vessels, and ligaments.

Immediate treatment

Wash any associated cuts to prevent infection and apply ice to reduce swelling. Elevate the injured hand and avoid using it.

Rehabilitation and prevention

Prevention of metacarpal fractures requires avoidance of activities likely to produce them, particularly striking hard objects with the hand. Preventing further injury to already fractured metacarpals is usually accomplished by immobilizing the hand, either with a finger splint or short cast, depending on the nature of the metacarpal fracture. Exercises designed to gradually increase movement, flexion, and extension of the wrist or fingers will help restore full use.

Long-term prognosis

Full recovery from most metacarpal fractures can be expected with aggressive early attention, which may include resetting of the bone and immobilization of the hand. Surgery may be required in the case of displaced bones, with the affected metacarpal realigned and held fast by means of removable pins.

020: THUMB SPRAIN (ULNAR COLLATERAL LIGAMENT)

Brief outline of injury

Many activities can pull the thumb suddenly away from the rest of the hand, stretching or occasionally tearing this ligament. The injury is very prevalent among skiers and is often referred to as *skier's thumb*, though repetitive activities that gradually wear and irritate the ulnar collateral ligament can produce a chronic form of injury.

Anatomy and physiology

A thumb sprain involves a fibrous band of tissue lying on either side of the thumb, known as the *ulnar collateral ligament*. The ulnar collateral ligament connects the metacarpal bone to the first phalanx at the base of the thumb (the thumb has two phalanges). Its function is to prevent the thumb from stretching too far away from the hand. The ligament is required for pinching and grasping activities.

Cause of injury

Thumb being jammed into another player, piece of equipment or the ground. Repetitive wear of the ulnar collateral ligament through gripping between the thumb and index finger. Any activity that violently separates the thumb from the rest of the hand, such as a skiing fall.

Signs and symptoms

Local pain and swelling over the torn ligament. Difficulty grasping objects or holding them firmly. Instability of the thumb which may repeatedly catch on objects or clothing.

Complications if left unattended

If a torn ulnar collateral ligament is left untreated, it may result in a painful, unstable thumb with loss of mobility. Continued soreness and a propensity for re-injury are also possible.

Immediate treatment

Elevation and ice for thirty minutes every two hours. Immobilize with a splint.

Rehabilitation and prevention

Buddy taping the thumb to its neighbouring digit, especially during contact sports, may help prevent re-injury. Gradual use of motion exercises to restore thumb movement should be undertaken as the ulnar collateral ligament undergoes final repair.

Long-term prognosis

Non-contact sports may usually be permitted six weeks following the injury, and a return to contact sports can be expected after three months, depending on the severity of the original sprain.

Rehabilitation exercises

021: MALLET FINGER (LONG EXTENSOR TENDON)

Brief outline of injury

Extensor tendons are vulnerable to injury, lying just below the skin surface directly on the bones of the back of the hand and fingers. Such tendons may be torn apart when a finger is jammed, separating the tendons from their attachment to bone. The injury is common at the start of baseball season, often caused by a ball hitting the fingertip, bending it sharply downward and tearing the extensor tendon. Cuts to the hand or fingers can also damage the extensor tendons.

Anatomy and physiology

Extensor tendons are small muscle tendons in the hand and fingers, which provide for delicate movements and hand coordination. They are located on the dorsal aspect of the hand and fingers, allowing the athlete to extend and straighten the fingers and thumb. Extensor tendons attach to muscles in the forearm. When an object hits the fingertip, the forceful flexion of the distal phalanx avulses the lateral bands of the extensor mechanism from its distal attachment.

Cause of injury

Cuts or lacerations affecting the extensor tendons. Baseball, volleyball, football, basketball or other object striking the fingertips while the extensor tendon is taut. Jamming the finger against a wall, door or other immovable object.

Signs and symptoms

Inability to extend the finger. Bruising, pain, and swelling of the affected finger. Drooping fingertip.

Complications if left unattended

Left untreated, mallet finger may cause permanent cosmetic deformity in the finger, though often without further complication. Without splinting however, some residual stiffness and loss of finger extension may result. Surgical intervention is typically not advised in simple cases of mallet finger as surgical complications may include stiffness, nail bed damage, infection, and chronic tenderness.

Immediate treatment

R.I.C.E.R. regimen for the first two days, followed by heat treatment. Immobilization with a splint pending medical consultation.

Rehabilitation and prevention

Generally, a splint must be worn continuously until the extensor tendon is fully healed. It will often require several months for local swelling and erythema to fully subside. Special care to the fingertips should always be taken in sports involving fast-moving balls, as well as when handling cutting implements.

Long-term prognosis

With attention to post-injury care including immobilization of the injured finger, most athletes achieve full restoration of movement and appearance of the digit.

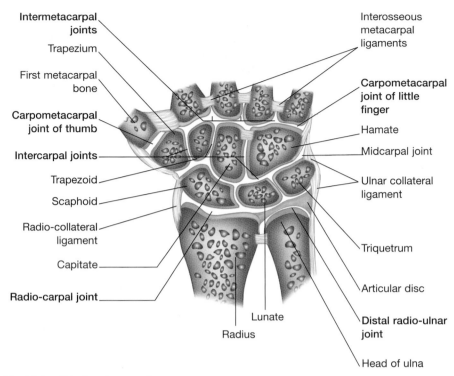

Intermetacarpal joints

Trapezium

First metacarpal bone

Carpometacarpal joint of thumb

Intercarpal joints

Trapezoid

Scaphoid

Radio-collateral ligament

Capitate

Radio-carpal joint

Interosseous metacarpal ligaments

Carpometacarpal joint of little finger

Hamate

Midcarpal joint

Ulnar collateral ligament

Triquetrum

Articular disc

Distal radio-ulnar joint

Head of ulna

Lunate

Radius

Figure 6.2: The joints of the hand, coronal view.

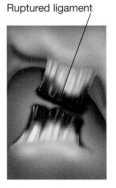

Ruptured ligament

Finger sprain

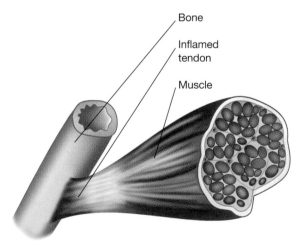

Bone

Inflamed tendon

Muscle

Hand/finger tendinitis

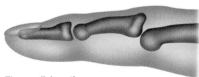

Finger dislocation

Rehabilitation exercises

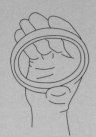

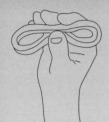

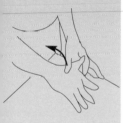

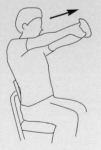

Brief outline of injury

Finger sprains are injuries to a joint that cause a stretch or tear in a ligament. Ligaments are resilient bands of tissue connecting one bone to another. Such sprains are common in a wide variety of sports including football, basketball, cricket, and handball. Such sprains include metacarpophalangeal and interphalangeal sprains, Boutonnière deformity, and mallet finger.

Anatomy and physiology

The fingers of the hand are composed of a number of joints, which are required to allow for the fine motor control of the fingers. The metacarpophalangeal (MCP)(knuckle) joints are condyloid joints, each of which is enclosed in a capsule that is reinforced by strong collateral ligaments. The carpometacarpal (CM) joint of the thumb is a saddle joint, and the carpometacarpal (CM) joints of the fingers are plane joints. The intermetacarpal (IM) joints are also plane joints, and both the CM and IM joints are surrounded by a joint capsule. The interphalangeal (IP) joints, both distal (DIP) and proximal (PIP), are hinge joints.

Injuries to the proximal interphalangeal (PIP) joint (the middle joint of the finger) are most common, and may result when the joint is straightened too far, (hyperextension). This can cause rupture or tearing of the *volar plate* (see page 82), a ligament connecting the proximal and middle phalanges to the collateral ligaments found on either side of the PIP joint.

Cause of injury

Blow to the hand at the region of the joint. Hyperextension of the joint, damaging the volar plate ligament. Collateral ligaments overstretched in a side to side displacement.

Signs and symptoms

Pain and tenderness in the finger. Pain when moving the finger joint. Swelling of the PIP finger joint, with deformity in the case of joint displacement.

Complications if left unattended

Should a deformity associated with finger sprain become chronic, the chances for surgical correction are reduced. Potential for permanent functional deficit in the injured finger exists.

Immediate treatment

Use of anti-inflammatory or other pain medication to reduce swelling. Applying ice packs to injured finger for 20–30 minutes every 3–4 hours for 2–3 days or until pain subsides.

Rehabilitation and prevention

Most finger sprain injuries, depending on severity, will be splinted or *buddy taped* to neighbouring digits in order to immobilize the area of trauma. Finger strains tend to be unforeseen and unpreventable injuries, though proper sports technique and equipment may reduce the likelihood of some sprains. Strengthening and mobility exercises for the fingers may be undertaken following initial healing.

Long-term prognosis

Full recovery and restoration of function in the injured finger is likely in most cases of finger sprains.

Brief outline of injury

Finger dislocations are more severe injuries than sprains and involve the displacement of the joint, altering the alignment of the finger. The joint must therefore be reset before the finger may be immobilized with casting, splint or taping. Splints allow the ligaments and joint capsule to properly heal. Such dislocations are common to many sports, particularly contact sports in which the athlete's hands come in direct physical contact with other players (football, wrestling) or other sports emphasizing use of the hands (volleyball, baseball, basketball, gymnastics, karate, and so forth).

Anatomy and physiology

Dislocation of a joint involves the tearing of ligaments and joint capsules surrounding the affected joint. Dislocation may occur in any of the joints in any of the fingers. Dislocation of the interphalangeal joints occurs most commonly in basketball and football. Dislocations of the metacarpophalangeal (MCP) and basilar carpometacarpal (CM) joints can occur during falls on the outstretched hand.

Cause of injury

Fingers being struck by a football, baseball, basketball, etc. Falling onto the outstretched hand. Abduction force applied to the thumb, as in a skier's fall.

Signs and symptoms

Immediate pain and swelling. Finger appears crooked. Inability to straighten or bend the dislocated joint.

Complications if left unattended

Deformity of the joint, loss of function, and developing arthritis can accompany an untreated finger dislocation. While some dislocations correct themselves without medical intervention, generally the displaced joint must be reset by a physician, followed by immobilization during the healing of the injury.

Immediate treatment

R.I.C.E.R. treatment should immediately follow the injury. Avoid all unnecessary movement of the injured finger.

Rehabilitation and prevention

Ligaments occasionally do not heal adequately following dislocation, and surgery may be required to repair damaged structures. Generally, finger dislocations are successfully treated by resetting the misaligned joint and holding the area rigid by means of a splint until thorough healing of the ligament and joint capsule has taken place. Stretching, strengthening, and mobility exercises may follow, to avoid stiffening or mobility loss in the affected joint.

Long-term prognosis

Most finger dislocations do not result in long-term finger deformity or loss of function, and a full recovery may be expected given aggressive early treatment.

Rehabilitation exercises

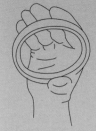
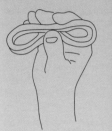
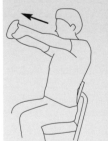
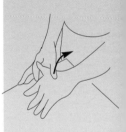

Rehabilitation exercises

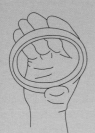

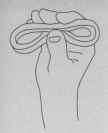

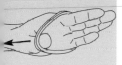

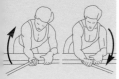

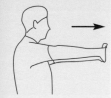

Brief outline of injury

Irritation and inflammation of tendons cause the condition of tendinitis, which may affect any of the tendons of the wrist or fingers. The affliction is common where overuse or overworking of the tendons is involved but can also be related to various underlying diseases, including *diabetes* and *rheumatoid arthritis.*

Anatomy and physiology

Tendons are resilient cords of tissue connecting muscle to bone, and act to transmit forces between the muscle and the skeleton, which requires them to bear considerable mechanical loads. Overworking of the tendons can lead to the inflammation of the tendons and tendon sheaths associated with tendinitis, which is often accompanied by *fibrinoid necrosis* and *myxomatous degeneration* (a condition where mucus accumulates in connective tissue).

Cause of injury

Intense or sustained exertion involving the tendons of the wrist or hand. Lack of adequate recovery time between athletic exertions. Cold temperatures or constant vibration in the hand.

Signs and symptoms

Tenderness. Inflammation. Crackling or grating sensation under the skin (crepitus).

Complications if left unattended

Should athletic activity continue despite existing tendinitis, the affliction can become chronic, and permanent damage to the structure of the tendons may result.

Immediate treatment

Anti-inflammatory drugs. Ice for the first 24–48 hours after onset of the condition.

Rehabilitation and prevention

Following rest and measures to reduce inflammation, strengthening and stretching exercises targeting the affected tendons can be undertaken, providing pain has subsided. Avoidance of repetitive stress to the tendons and ensuring proper recovery times following physical activities involving the wrist and hands can help prevent recurrence of the condition.

Long-term prognosis

Proper care of tendinitis usually results in reduction of inflammation, alleviation of pain and full recovery of movement, though the condition can become chronic, particularly in elite athletes, whose schedule demands repeated overstress of tendons.

Chapter 7

Sports Injuries of the
Wrists and Forearm

Acute

025: Wrist and Forearm Fracture

026: Wrist Sprain

027: Wrist Dislocation

Chronic

028: Carpal Tunnel Syndrome

029: Ulnar Tunnel Syndrome

030: Wrist Ganglion Cyst

031: Wrist Tendinitis

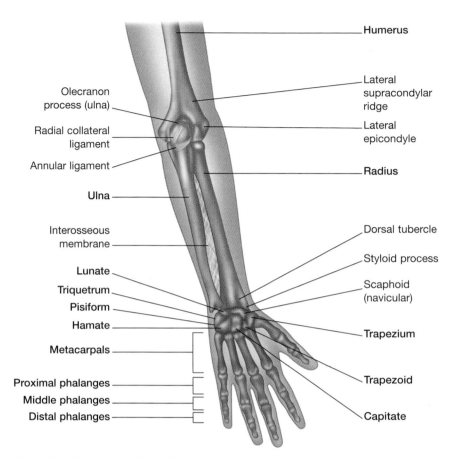

Olecranon process (ulna)

Radial collateral ligament

Annular ligament

Ulna

Interosseous membrane

Lunate

Triquetrum

Pisiform

Hamate

Metacarpals

Proximal phalanges

Middle phalanges

Distal phalanges

Humerus

Lateral supracondylar ridge

Lateral epicondyle

Radius

Dorsal tubercle

Styloid process

Scaphoid (navicular)

Trapezium

Trapezoid

Capitate

Figure 7.1: The bones of the right forearm and hand, posterior view.

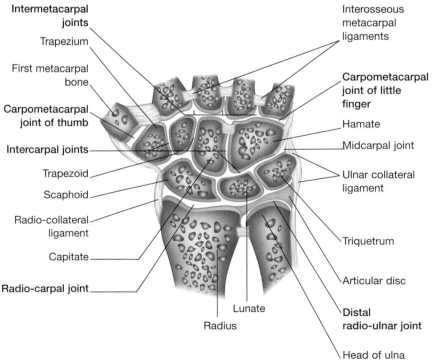

Intermetacarpal joints

Trapezium

First metacarpal bone

Carpometacarpal joint of thumb

Intercarpal joints

Trapezoid

Scaphoid

Radio-collateral ligament

Capitate

Radio-carpal joint

Interosseous metacarpal ligaments

Carpometacarpal joint of little finger

Hamate

Midcarpal joint

Ulnar collateral ligament

Triquetrum

Articular disc

Distal radio-ulnar joint

Head of ulna

Lunate

Radius

Figure 7.1a: The joints of the wrist and hand, coronal view.

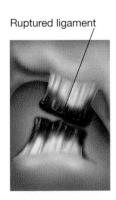

Ruptured ligament

Wrist sprain

Brief outline of injury

Should an athlete fall on an outstretched wrist, a break or fracture of the wrist or bones of the forearm may result. Sports vulnerable to such injury include running, cycling, skateboarding, rollerblading and other activities in which an outstretched hand may be used to break a fall.

Anatomy and physiology

The wrist consists of a series of radio-carpal and intercarpal articulations. However, most wrist movement occurs at the radio-carpal joint, an ellipsoid joint. The distal surface of the radius and the articular disc articulate with the proximal row of carpals: the *scaphoid*, *lunate*, and *triquestral* (triquetrum). Movements are in combination with the intercarpal joints. The intercarpal joints are a series of plane joints, which have articulations between the two carpal rows (midcarpal joint), plus articulations between each bone of the proximal carpal row and of the distal carpal row. The distal radio-ulnar joint is immediately adjacent to the radio-carpal joint. A cartilaginous disc separates the distal ulna and radius from the lunate and triquetral bones. Wrist fractures are breaks in one or more of these bones. The two most common wrist fractures are *Colles' fracture*, which occurs near the end of the radius, and *scaphoid fracture*, which involves the *scaphoid* or *navicular*, a small bone located on the thumb-side of the wrist that joins the radius.

Cause of injury

A fall onto an outstretched wrist. A blow to the wrist. Extreme twisting of the wrist.

Signs and symptoms

Deformity of the wrist. Pain and swelling. Limited motion in the thumb or wrist.

Complications if left unattended

Wrist fractures often fuse naturally, though complications may arise in the untreated fracture leading to limitations of wrist movement and forearm rotation, pronation, and supination. Osteoarthritis may also arise following untreated fractures. Untreated or misdiagnosed scaphoid fractures run the risk of non-union or malunion of fractured bone segments.

Immediate treatment

Apply an ice pack over the wrist to reduce swelling. Elevate the fractured wrist or forearm and place it in a sling.

Rehabilitation and prevention

Immobilization with a rigid cast is generally required for such fractures to properly heal, with x-ray follow-ups to analyze improvement. Where surgery is required, wires or screws may be employed to fuse fractured segments.

Long-term prognosis

Prognosis in the case of radius or ulna fractures depends on the complication of the fracture patterns. Open fractures (where the skin is broken) tend to have less favorable outcomes. Most scaphoid fractures of the wrist heal thoroughly if immobilized early after injury and allowed to heal for 8–12 weeks.

Brief outline of injury

Wrist sprains involve injury to the ligaments of the wrist. Such sprains are a common occurrence when the hand is extended to break a fall. Ligaments are necessary for stabilization of the hand and control of motion. Wrist sprains vary from moderate to severe, with the latter involving complete tearing of the ligaments and instability of the accompanying joint. The injury is common to athletes engaged in football, basketball, skiing, snowboarding, rollerblading, and a variety of other sports in which the hands are vulnerable.

Anatomy and physiology

The eight carpal bones of the wrist are connected together via ligaments—fibrous bands of tissue. Such ligaments also connect the bones of the wrist with the radius, ulna, and metacarpal bones. The smooth coordination of these bones required for proper hand movement is impaired when one or more ligaments are injured.

Cause of injury

Engaging in sports where falls are common, e.g. in-line skating, snowboarding, cycling, soccer, football, baseball, and volleyball. Lack of protective equipment, including wrist guards. Muscle weakness or atrophy.

Signs and symptoms

Pain with movement of the wrist. Burning or tingling feeling at the wrist. Bruising or discolouration of the skin.

Complications if left unattended

Moderate to severe wrist sprains left untreated can lead to ongoing deficit of movement and strength in the wrist as well as developing arthritis at the region of the injury.

Immediate treatment

R.I.C.E.R. regimen immediately following injury. Immobilization of injured wrist to restrict movement.

Rehabilitation and prevention

Flexibility and range of motion exercises may be encouraged by a physical therapist, following initial recovery of the ligament. Should the ligament be torn completely, or if fracture accompanies the sprain, surgery may be required. Use of protective guards for wrists and concentration on balance during sport may help to avoid this injury.

Long-term prognosis

Most wrist sprains undergo full recovery given proper initial care and necessary healing time.

Rehabilitation exercises

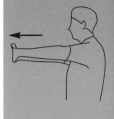
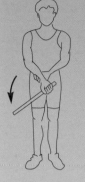
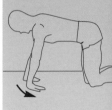
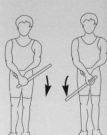
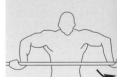

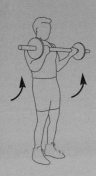

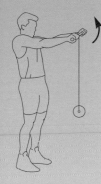

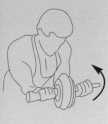

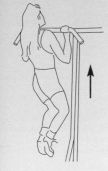

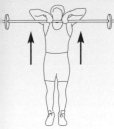

Brief outline of injury

Most dislocations of the wrist involve the lunate bone, though other bones may also be involved. When a bone is dislocated, it no longer properly makes contact with adjoining bones. The injury affects the soft tissue surrounding the region of dislocation, including muscles, nerves, tendons, ligaments, and blood vessels.

Anatomy and physiology

The wrist consists of a series of radio-carpal and intercarpal articulations. However, most wrist movement occurs at the *radio-carpal joint*, an ellipsoid joint. The distal surface of the radius and the articular disc articulates with the proximal row of carpals, which are the *scaphoid, lunate,* and *triquestral* (triquetrum). Movements are in combination with the *intercarpal joints.* The intercarpal joints are a series of plane joints, which have articulations between the two carpal rows (midcarpal joint), plus articulations between each bone of the proximal carpal row and of the distal carpal row. The distal radio-ulnar joint is immediately adjacent to the radio-carpal joint. A cartilaginous disc separates the distal ulna and radius from the lunate and triquetral bones. An elaborate complex of ligaments holds these bones together and allows for their proper coordination. *Dorsal ligaments* of the wrist are weaker and more likely to be involved in dislocations.

Cause of injury

Complication of a severe wrist sprain. Hard fall on an outstretched hand. Congenital abnormality, including malformed joint surfaces.

Signs and symptoms

Loss of hand and wrist movement. Severe pain in the wrist. Numbness or paralysis below the dislocation due to severed blood vessels or nerves.

Complications if left unattended

Outcomes for untreated wrist dislocation are largely unpredictable, with some cases of full recovery and restoration of movement. Complications however may restrict motion of the wrist and produce ongoing pain, joint stiffness, discomfort, and impaired flexibility and movement. Arthritis may also develop in the injured region.

Immediate treatment

Immobilize the wrist and use R.I.C.E.R.

Rehabilitation and prevention

Exercises designed to strengthen wrist muscles and ligaments will help prevent re-injury. Protection of the wrist during athletics, with gloves, wrist guards or taping may also offer some protection against wrist dislocations.

Long-term prognosis

Prognosis depends on the severity of the dislocation and any attendant complications, including fracture. Proper early treatment and appropriate rehabilitation leads to full recovery in most cases.

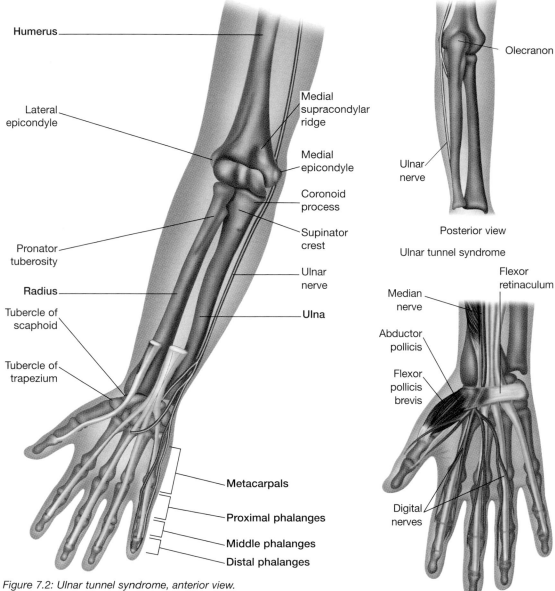

Humerus

Lateral
epicondyle

Medial
supracondylar
ridge

Medial
epicondyle

Coronoid
process

Supinator
crest

Pronator
tuberosity

Ulnar
nerve

Radius

Ulna

Tubercle of
scaphoid

Tubercle of
trapezium

Metacarpals

Proximal phalanges

Middle phalanges

Distal phalanges

Olecranon

Ulnar
nerve

Posterior view

Ulnar tunnel syndrome

Flexor
retinaculum

Median
nerve

Abductor
pollicis

Flexor
pollicis
brevis

Digital
nerves

Carpal tunnel syndrome

Figure 7.2: Ulnar tunnel syndrome, anterior view.

Ulnar artery
Ulnar nerve
Flexor digitorum
superficialis tendons
Carpal tunnel
Flexor digitorum
profundus tendons
Extensor carpi ulnaris tendon
Extensor digiti minimi tendon
Basilic vein
Extensor digitorum tendons

Palmaris longus tendon
Flexor retinaculum
Median nerve
Flexor carpi radialis tendon
Flexor pollicis longus tendon
Abductor pollicis longus tendon
Extensor pollicis brevis tendon
Cephalic vein
Radial artery
Extensor carpi
radialis longus tendon
Extensor pollicis longus tendon
Extensor carpi radialis
brevis tendon
Extensor indicis tendon

Cross-section of the wrist

Rehabilitation exercises

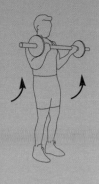

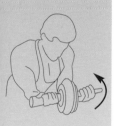

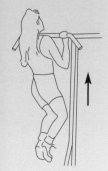

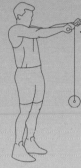

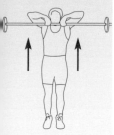

Brief outline of injury

Carpal tunnel syndrome (CTS) is a progressive affliction caused by direct trauma or repetitive overuse, which results in squeezing or compression of the median nerve at the wrist. The condition is three times more likely to affect women, largely due to occupational tasks such as keyboard work.

Anatomy and physiology

The carpal tunnel is a narrow, rigid structure composed of ligament and bone at the base of the hand. This nerve runs from the forearm to the hand and transmits sensations from the palm side of the thumb and fingers, as well as impulses to certain small muscles of the hand involved in movement. The tunnel surrounds the *median nerve* (which enters the hand between the carpal bones), and *tendons*. A narrowing of the tunnel may occur as a result of irritated or inflamed tendons, leading to pressure and compression of the median nerve, causing pain, weakness or numbness in the hand, which gradually radiates up the arm. The condition is one of a variety of *entrapment neuropathies*—afflictions involving compression or trauma to peripheral nerves.

Cause of injury

Sporting activities that involve repetitive flexion and extension of the wrist, e.g. cycling, throwing events, racket sports, and gymnastics. Congenital predisposition. Trauma or injury including fracture or sprain. Occupational tasks.

Signs and symptoms

Burning, numbness or itching in the palm of the hand and fingers. Sensation of finger and wrist swelling. Decreased grip strength. Pain that may wake the individual during the night.

Complications if left unattended

Left untreated, carpal tunnel syndrome can lead to decreased or absent sensation in some fingers and permanent weakness of the thumb, as muscles of the thumb degenerate. Proper sensation of hot and cold temperatures may also be diminished in untreated CTS cases.

Immediate treatment

Cease repetitive stress activity causing the condition. Immobilization of the wrist with bandage or splint to prevent further irritation.

Rehabilitation and prevention

Halting the repetitive sport or activity and allowing for rest and rehabilitation time following diagnosis of carpal tunnel syndrome is essential. A bandage or splint may be used to stabilize the injured hand. Releasing the tension in the wrist and hand during sports and periodic exercises to retain mobility and retard stiffness in the hands may help prevent the onset of CTS.

Long-term prognosis

Recurrence of carpal tunnel syndrome following treatment is rare, (except in cases of underlying disease, diabetes, endocrine disorders, etc.). The majority of patients properly attending to the injury recover completely.

029: ULNAR TUNNEL SYNDROME

Brief outline of injury

One of three major nerves responsible for motor function and sensation in the hand, the ulnar nerve runs along the inside of the forearm, reaching down to the heel of the hand. In the hand, the ulnar nerve radiates across the palm and into the little finger and ring finger. Pressure on the ulnar nerve can result in pain, loss of sensation and muscle weakness in the hand.

Anatomy and physiology

The humerus of the upper arm has three bony points, frequently associated with repetitive strain injuries. Two of these bony points are involved in ulnar tunnel syndrome, the *olecranon* and the *medial epicondyle* in the elbow. The space between these bony protrusions is known as the *ulnar tunnel*. The ulnar nerve, which acts on the muscle that pulls the thumb toward the palm of the hand, also controls small *intrinsic* muscles of the hand. It passes through the *cubital* or *ulnar tunnel* at the elbow, running down the forearm and into the hand. It is one of the three major nerves in the arm, the others being the *radial* and *median nerves*.

Cause of injury

Overuse of muscles and tendons of the forearm, especially in golf, and sports involving throwing. Abnormal growth in the wrist, such as a cyst. Sudden trauma to the ulnar nerve within the ulnar tunnel.

Signs and symptoms

Weakness and increasing numbness on the little finger side of the hand. Difficulty grasping and holding objects. Tingling along the outer forearm, especially when the elbow is bent.

Complications if left unattended

Without proper treatment, ulnar tunnel syndrome can lead to permanent nerve damage and chronic weakening and numbness, due to reduced blood supply to the ulnar nerve when the elbow is bent.

Immediate treatment

Cease the activity which is causing pressure on the ulnar nerve, and avoid keeping the elbow in a bent position. Splint or pad, especially at night to keep the arm straight.

Rehabilitation and prevention

In the case of ulnar tunnel syndrome due to an abnormal growth such as a cyst, surgery may be required to remove it. Where repetitive stress or exercise have led to ulnar nerve inflammation, non-surgical physical therapy, including strengthening exercises will often yield improvement in 4–6 weeks. A pad or splint may be used to reduce symptoms at night.

Long-term prognosis

In cases where ulnar tunnel syndrome receives prompt and appropriate attention, the prognosis for full recovery is good. Nerve damage and deficit can result however, should the condition be allowed to persist without care.

Rehabilitation exercises

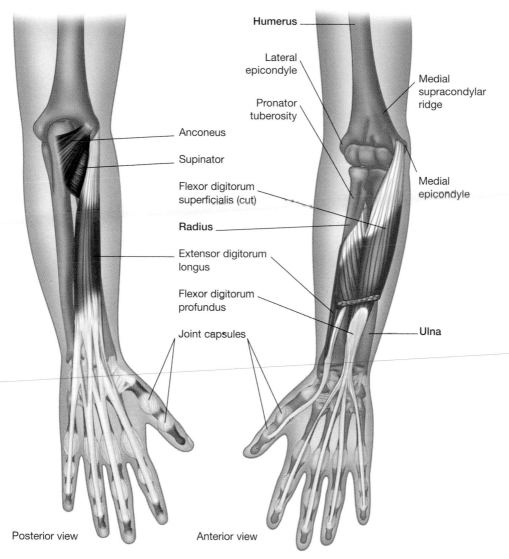

Humerus

Lateral
epicondyle

Medial
supracondylar
ridge

Pronator
tuberosity

Anconeus

Supinator

Medial
epicondyle

Flexor digitorum
superficialis (cut)

Radius

Extensor digitorum
longus

Flexor digitorum
profundus

Joint capsules

Ulna

Posterior view

Anterior view

Figure 5.4: Right forearm, wrist and hand.

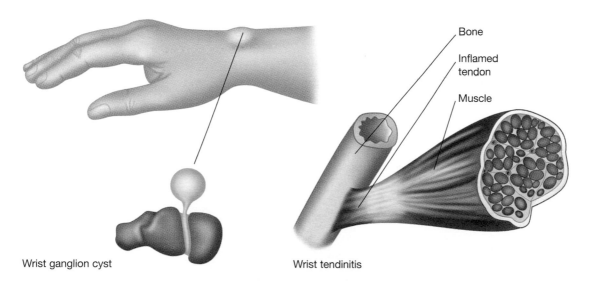

Bone

Inflamed
tendon

Muscle

Wrist ganglion cyst

Wrist tendinitis

Brief outline of injury

A ganglion (Greek: knot of tissue) cyst is a bump or mass that forms under the skin. They can occur at any joint or tendon sheath, but most often on the back of the wrist or on the fingers. Ganglion cysts are probably the most common lumps that occur in the hand. Most often, ganglion cysts occur in the 25–45 year old age group, and they are more common in women than they are in men. Ganglion cysts are benign tumours (so do not spread to other body areas), and their cause is unknown. Sometimes they are also called *synovial hernias* or *synovial cysts* because of their relationship to the synovial cavities in the joint. Also known as *subchondral cysts*.

Anatomy and physiology

Ganglion cysts are thin, fibrous capsules containing a clear, mucinous fluid, and feel soft and moveable. Ganglion cysts have a smooth translucent wall, generally connected to an underlying joint capsule or ligament via a thin stalk. Ganglion cysts can involve any joint in the hand or wrist, mainly occur on an *aponeurosis* or *tendon*, and are palpable between the extensor tendons. The ganglion cyst forms when tissue around the joint becomes inflamed and swells with fluid. As this happens, the balloon-like ganglion grows in the connective tissue of the joint or even in the membrane that covers the nearby tendon. Often, cysts are associated with the scapholunate ligament or scaphotrapezial joint of the wrist. Most cysts occur at the dorsal wrist, volar wrist, and volar retinacular or distal interphalangeal area.

Cause of injury

Flaw in the joint capsule. Flaw in the tendon sheath. Tissue trauma.

Signs and symptoms

Swollen sac-like area, which changes size. May or may not produce pain. Wrist weakness.

Complications if left unattended

Most ganglion cysts disappear without treatment, though in some cases, they recur over time. Such cysts generally do not pose a serious health risk, even if left untreated, though pain and weakness of the wrist may persist without medical care.

Immediate treatment

Ice three times a day if the cyst is painful. Aspirin or anti-inflammatory medication.

Rehabilitation and prevention

Cysts may be drained of fluid by a physician. The patient should not attempt this. Often, cysts will gradually disappear without draining or surgical intervention, though they may recur. If the ganglion cyst is painful, sports involving intensive use of the wrist should be limited or avoided until shrinkage or disappearance of the cyst.

Long-term prognosis

Cysts may be asymptomatic and self-limiting. Should medical attention be required, the prognosis for full recovery is excellent.

Rehabilitation exercises

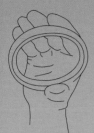

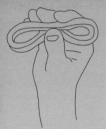

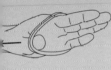

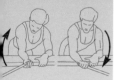

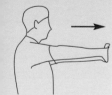

Brief outline of injury

Wrist tendinitis is due to irritation and inflammation of one or more tendons around the wrist joint. Wrist tendinitis tends to occur in areas where the tendons cross each other or pass over an underlying bony structure, and affects individuals involved in strenuous and repetitive training.

Anatomy and physiology

The joint of the wrist is formed at the proximal end by the distal surfaces of the radius and ulna and a disc of fibrocartilage, and at the distal end by the scaphoid, lunate, and triquetral bones. The wrist helps orient and support the hand. Tendons of the wrist are encased in tendon sheaths known as the *tenosynovium*. Such sheaths provide for the smooth, friction-free sliding of tendons in the wrist. Swelling, irritation, and inflammation of the tenosynovium causes a thickening of the sheath, which constricts proper movement of the tendons, resulting in pain and a related affliction, *tenosynovitis*. Most wrist tendinitis occurs where a tendon passes through constricted tunnels of fascia. Four common sites of tendinitis are the first dorsal compartment (De Quervain's tendovaginitis), digital flexors (trigger finger), flexor carpi radialis tendinitis, and lateral epicondylitis, (the latter associated with tennis elbow). The abductor pollicis longus and extensor pollicis brevis are also commonly affected.

Cause of injury

Sports involving wrist overuse, including all ball sports, racquet sports, rowing, weightlifting, gymnastics, etc. Repetitive stress from typing. Other wrist overuse, as is common to nursing mothers.

Signs and symptoms

Pain in the wrist, particularly at the joint. Inflammation in the region of the affected tendon(s). Limited mobility in the affected wrist.

Complications if left unattended

If the activity causing tendinitis is continued and the condition left untreated, the inflammation and associated pain can worsen. The condition can also lead to permanent weakening of the tendon(s).

Immediate treatment

Immobilize the wrist and use R.I.C.E.R. Anti-inflammatory medication.

Rehabilitation and prevention

Often, a physician will use a splint or brace to prevent movement of the injured wrist. In athletic events, tendinitis sometimes results from improper technique. The best therapy for tendinitis is to restrict or temporarily discontinue the activity causing tendon inflammation.

Long-term prognosis

Most enjoy a full recovery from tendinitis, providing the afflicted wrist is permitted proper recuperation from inflammation.

Chapter

8

Sports Injuries of the
Elbow

Acute

032: Elbow Fracture

033: Elbow Sprain

034: Elbow Dislocation

035: Triceps Brachii Tendon Rupture

Chronic

036: Tennis Elbow

037: Golfer's Elbow

038: Thrower's Elbow

039: Elbow Bursitis

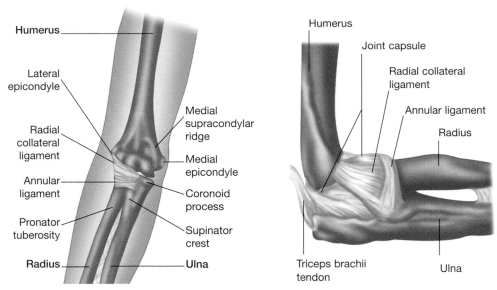

Figure 8.1: The elbow joint, anterior view.

Figure 8.2: The elbow joint, right arm, lateral view.

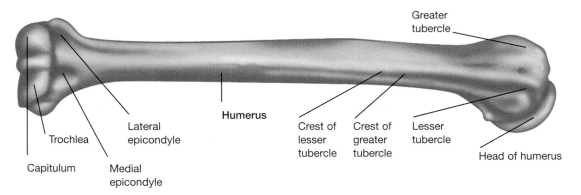

Figure 8.3: The right humerus, anterior view.

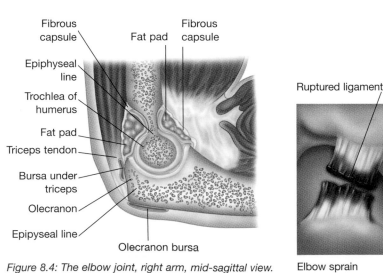

Figure 8.4: The elbow joint, right arm, mid-sagittal view.

Elbow sprain

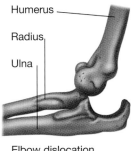

Elbow dislocation

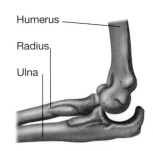

Elbow subluxation

Rehabilitation exercises

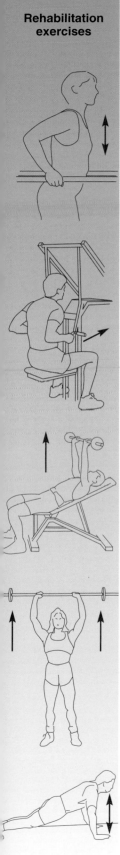

Brief outline of injury

An elbow fracture is a break involving any of the three arm bones that work together to form the elbow joint. Such fractures may occur as the result of a blunt force striking the elbow during athletics or from a fall on the elbow. The injury is common to many sports, particularly contact sports such as football. Fractures may be classified as *distal humeral fractures, radial fractures,* and *ulnar fractures.* Fractures of the *radial head* are the most common.

Anatomy and physiology

The elbow is a hinge joint that is comprised of three bones, the upper arm bone or *humerus*, and the two bones of the forearm, the *ulna* and the *radius*. Of the forearm bones, the ulna is the most medial, being on the little finger side, and also the largest. At the distal end of the humerus, are the *trochlea* and the *capitulum*, which form part of the elbow joint with the radius and ulna. The *annular ligament* binds the head of the radius to the ulna, forming the *proximal radio-ulnar joint.*

Cause of injury

Falling directly onto the elbow. Direct trauma to the elbow. Severe torsion of the elbow beyond its normal range of motion.

Signs and symptoms

Swelling and pain in the region of the elbow. Deformity of the elbow due to bone fracture. Loss of arm mobility.

Complications if left unattended

Without treatment, fractured bones of the elbow can fail to heal properly, and at times, fuse in misalignment. This can lead to long-term deficit in arm motion and strength, increased vulnerability to re-injury, and deformity of the joint.

Immediate treatment

Apply ice immediately to the swollen area. Immobilize the arm in a splint or sling before seeking emergency help.

Rehabilitation and prevention

Elbow fractures occur from sudden, accidental trauma and are often difficult to prevent. Avoiding athletics at periods of extreme fatigue and protection of the elbow with padding during athletics are both prudent. Additionally, consuming calcium and performing bone strengthening exercises may help avoid fractures.

Long-term prognosis

Long-term prospects for elbow fractures vary depending on the nature and severity of the fracture as well as the age and medical history of the injured athlete. Infections, stiffening of the elbow joint, arthritis, non-union or malunion of bone are possible. In the case of less severe elbow fractures, full recovery may be expected, though the healing process often requires several months.

Brief outline of injury

Ligaments are strong bands of tissue connecting bones and crossing joints, and act to stabilize the elbow. A sprain involves the stretching or tearing of elbow ligaments. Many sports are prone to elbow sprains, particularly sports involving throwing, and often involve the medial collateral ligament. Elbow sprains are also common in gymnastics.

Anatomy and physiology

The elbow contains several important ligaments, the two most important being the *ulnar (medial) collateral ligament* and the *radial (lateral) collateral ligament*. The ulnar (medial) collateral ligament is composed of three strong bands that reinforce the medial side of the capsule. The radial (lateral) collateral ligament is a strong triangular ligament that reinforces the lateral side of the capsule. These ligaments connect the humerus bone to the ulna and act together to stabilize the elbow. Additionally, the *annular ligament* envelopes the head of the radius bone and holds it firmly against the ulna.

Cause of injury

Sudden, abnormal twisting of the arm. Falling on an outstretched arm. Deficient strength in arm ligaments and muscles.

Signs and symptoms

Pain, tenderness, and swelling in the area of the elbow joint. Bruising around the elbow. Limited range of motion in the arm.

Complications if left unattended

Sprains, particularly when they are severe, can lead to future painful or disabling symptoms, including instability and weakness in the elbow, limited range of motion and occasionally, osteoarthritis.

Immediate treatment

R.I.C.E.R. regimen to reduce inflammation and treat pain. Immobilization of injured elbow with a sling or splint.

Rehabilitation and prevention

Proper athletic technique, avoiding exercise during periods of fatigue, and protective sportswear including padding can all reduce the risk of elbow sprains. Following initial healing, range of motion exercises and gradual return to athletic activity will help restore flexibility. Often for a time however, a supportive brace may be used to prevent sudden re-injury.

Long-term prognosis

Depending on the severity of the sprain and general health of the patient, minor sprains heal thoroughly without future complication. Older athletes or those who have suffered severe sprain (including sprains occurring in conjunction with fractures or dislocations), may suffer some impairment of movement and pain associated with arthritis.

Rehabilitation exercises

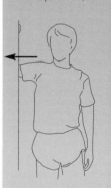

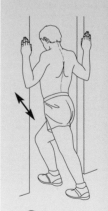

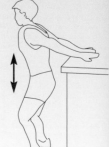

034: ELBOW DISLOCATION

Rehabilitation exercises

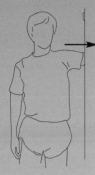

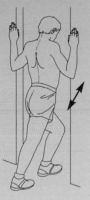

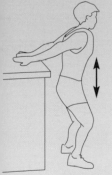

Brief outline of injury

Dislocation of the elbow occurs when the upper arm bone or *humerus*, moves out of place from the two bones of the forearm, the *ulna* and *radius*. The three bones meet at the elbow joint, which is displaced in an elbow dislocation. The injury typically produces considerable pain, swellings and loss of movement in the injured arm. Contact sports are more prone to such injuries. Fractures as well as injuries to arteries and nerves sometimes accompany dislocation. A *partial* dislocation is known as a *subluxation*.

Anatomy and physiology

The elbow provides the arm with flexion and extension capacity as well as pronation and supination ability, affording great range of motion. Considerable force is required to dislocate the elbow hinge joint. The humerus and ulna are generally stable and are reinforced by ligaments, primarily the *ulnar (medial) collateral ligament*, which is composed of three strong bands (anterior oblique, posterior oblique, and transverse) that reinforce the medial side of the capsule. The *radial (lateral) collateral ligament* is a strong triangular ligament that reinforces the lateral side of the capsule. These ligaments connect the humerus to the ulna and act together to stabilize the elbow.

Cause of injury

Blow or other trauma to the elbow. Fall onto an outstretched arm. Violent contact between the elbow and another athlete or object.

Signs and symptoms

Severe pain in the elbow, swelling, and loss of arm flexibility. Loss of feeling in the hand, following sharp injury to the elbow. Nerve or arterial injury following trauma to the elbow.

Complications if left unattended

Improper healing can follow a dislocation if left untreated. The results can involve nerve and arterial damage, osteoarthritis, ongoing pain in the injured arm, loss of full movement, and distortion of the elbow joint. Infection of the dislocated region is also possible, particularly if a fracture is involved.

Immediate treatment

Check for possible damage to an artery by taking the pulse. Treat the injury with ice and immobilize the elbow in a splint or sling.

Rehabilitation and prevention

Ice should be used to reduce initial pain and swelling, as proper medical attention is sought. The elbow should be moved as little as possible, and elevated frequently. Proper attention to athletic technique and padding of the elbow region, especially in the case of contact events like football, may help prevent such injuries.

Long-term prognosis

Generally, dislocations without further complication of nerve or artery damage, heal thoroughly given proper initial care and some rehabilitative exercises.

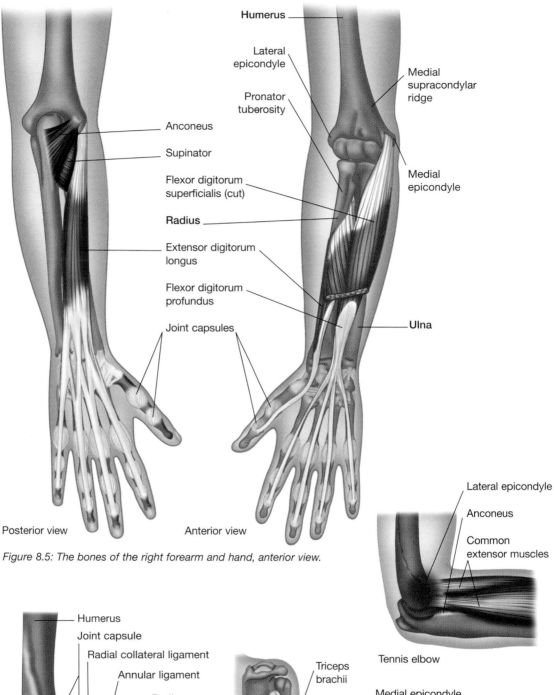

Humerus

Lateral epicondyle

Medial supracondylar ridge

Pronator tuberosity

Anconeus

Supinator

Medial epicondyle

Flexor digitorum superficialis (cut)

Radius

Extensor digitorum longus

Flexor digitorum profundus

Joint capsules

Ulna

Posterior view

Anterior view

Figure 8.5: The bones of the right forearm and hand, anterior view.

Lateral epicondyle

Anconeus

Common extensor muscles

Tennis elbow

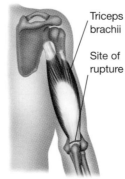

Triceps brachii

Site of rupture

Triceps brachii tendon rupture

Humerus

Joint capsule

Radial collateral ligament

Annular ligament

Radius

Triceps brachii tendon

Ulna

Figure 8.6: The elbow joint, right arm, lateral view.

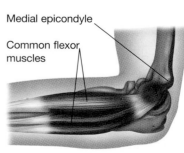

Medial epicondyle

Common flexor muscles

Golfer's elbow

Rehabilitation exercises

Brief outline of injury

The triceps brachii tendon is located at the back of the upper arm, inserting into the back of the elbow. A direct fall onto an outstretched hand can rupture this tendon (also known as *tendon avulsion*), though the injury is fairly uncommon. Weightlifters and football linemen are among the athletes who run a risk of triceps brachii tendon rupture, due to excessive weight on the tendon.

Anatomy and physiology

The triceps brachii tendon connects the ulna with the large triceps brachii muscle at the back of the arm. The tendon permits the elbow to straighten with force, during certain activities, e.g. push-ups. The tendon begins around the middle of the triceps brachii muscle and consists of two segments, one covering the back of the lower half of the muscle, the other, more deeply situated within the muscle. The two segments or *lamellæ* join each other above the elbow and insert into the olecranon.

Cause of injury

Fall on an outstretched hand, with the elbow in mid-flexion. Excessive weight lifting. Underlying health issues, such as *hyperparathyroidism* or *diabetes mellitus*.

Signs and symptoms

Pain and swelling in the elbow region. Limited mobility of the elbow. Muscle spasms.

Complications if left unattended

The injury generally requires surgery to repair. Failure to repair a ruptured triceps brachii tendon can cause permanent tendon deficiency, leading to muscle weakness, continued pain, and loss of arm mobility and weight bearing capacity.

Immediate treatment

R.I.C.E.R. regimen to reduce inflammation and treat pain. Prevent movement by immobilizing the injury with a splint or sling.

Rehabilitation and prevention

Following surgery to repair a ruptured triceps brachii tendon, exercises may be used to gradually increase the range of motion, flexibility, and strength of the injured arm. Proper technique, particularly if weightlifting or bodybuilding is critical to prevent such injuries. It is believed the use of *anabolic steroids* increases the risk of such tendon ruptures.

Long-term prognosis

With surgery soon after the time of injury and proper rehabilitation, ruptures of the triceps brachii tendon generally heal completely, though complications including accompanying fractures, etc. must be weighed up in assessing long-term outlook.

Brief outline of injury

Tennis elbow, also known as *lateral epicondylitis*, is the most common overuse injury in the adult elbow, and causes the outer part of the elbow to become painful and tender. The affliction is usually related to either overuse of the muscles attached to bone at the elbow, or, less frequently, direct trauma to the elbow. Often, extensor muscles of the hand, which attach at the elbow, become strained from overuse, causing inflammation and pain.

Anatomy and physiology

Tendons attached to the bones of the elbow can become restricted or taut, causing irritation. The *lateral epicondyle* is a bony attachment located on the top of the forearm, near the elbow. Various muscles attach to the lateral epicondyle, including the *anconeus* and *supinator* muscles, involved in rotating the forearm to the palm up position. Strain or overuse of extensor muscles (which lift the wrist away from the palm), can also cause tennis elbow.

Cause of injury

Overuse of the muscles attached to the elbow. Direct injury to the elbow. Arthritis, rheumatism, or gout.

Signs and symptoms

Outer part of the elbow is painful and tender to touch. Movement is painful. Elbow is inflamed.

Complications if left unattended

Tennis elbow is generally treated without surgery, though discomfort will often worsen with the potential for tendon or muscle damage, should the condition be ignored.

Immediate treatment

Avoidance of the activities causing repetitive stress to the elbow. R.I.C.E.R. regimen for 48–72 hours following injury. Use of anti-inflammatory drugs and analgesics.

Rehabilitation and prevention

Often, a splint or bandage will be used to immobilize the injured elbow and prevent excess movement. Activities involving repetitive stress to the elbow or extensor muscles of the wrist should be avoided until the condition improves. Should surgery be required, a rest period of six weeks is advised before strengthening exercises begin.

Long-term prognosis

Few patients suffering from tennis elbow require surgery, and of the small percentage that do, between 80% and 90% find the condition markedly improved.

Rehabilitation exercises

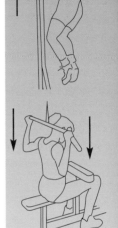

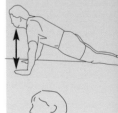

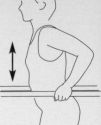

Rehabilitation exercises

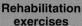

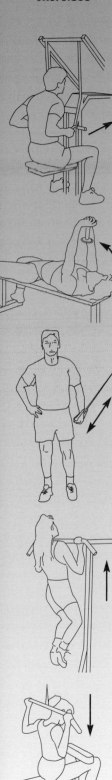

Brief outline of injury

Golfer's elbow, also known as *medial epicondylitis*, is a form of tendinitis similar to tennis elbow. Golfing is one of many sources of the affliction, which can result from any activity leading to overuse of the muscles and tendons of the forearm. While the painful sensation at the elbow is similar to tennis elbow, in the case of golfer's elbow, the pain and inflammation occur at the inside (or medial side) of the elbow around the bony prominence of the joint.

Anatomy and physiology

The *medial epicondyle* is a bony prominence on the inside of the elbow. It is the insertion point for muscles used to bend the wrist downward. Forceful, repetitive bending of the fingers and wrist can lead to small ruptures of muscle and tendon in this area. While the golfing swing produces a tightening in the flexor muscles and tendons that can lead to medial epicondylitis, other activities can produce the same injury.

Cause of injury

Sudden trauma or blow to the elbow. Repetitive stress to the flexor muscles and tendons of the wrist. Repeated stress placed on the arm during the acceleration phase of the throwing motion. Underlying health issues including neck problems, rheumatism, arthritis or gout.

Signs and symptoms

Tenderness and pain at the medial epicondyle, which worsens when the wrist is flexed. Pain resulting from lifting or grasping objects. Difficulty extending the forearm due to inflammation.

Complications if left unattended

Golfer's elbow, while generally alleviated by proper rest, can cause increasing pain and unpleasantness if the stressful activity continues. The condition rarely requires surgery, and responds well to proper rehabilitation. Should surgery be required, scar tissue is removed from the elbow where the tendons attach.

Immediate treatment

Avoidance of the activities causing repetitive stress to the elbow. R.I.C.E.R. regimen for 48–72 hours following the injury. Use of anti-inflammatory drugs and analgesics.

Rehabilitation and prevention

In the case of golfing, the affliction can be reduced in severity or prevented altogether through attention to proper technique and attention to overuse. Golfer's elbow is more prevalent early in the golf season, when muscles and tendons are not yet sufficiently conditioned. Rehabilitation generally involves avoiding the painful activity for a period. Use of analgesics for pain and anti-inflammatory drugs help reduce symptoms. After healing, resistive exercises may be undertaken to improve strength.

Long-term prognosis

Those suffering from golfer's elbow generally make a full recovery without surgery or advanced medical care, providing the injured elbow is afforded proper rest from the stressful activity.

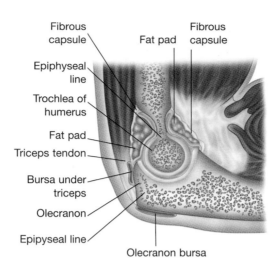

Figure 8.7: The elbow joint, right arm, mid-sagittal view.

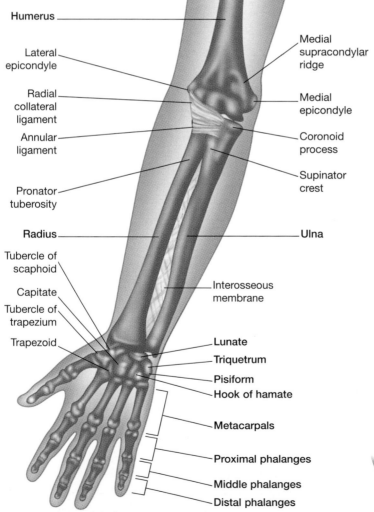

Figure 8.8: The bones of the right forearm and hand, anterior view.

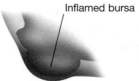

Elbow bursitis

Rehabilitation exercises

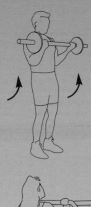

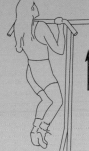

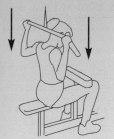

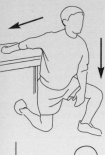

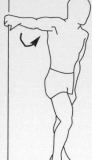

Brief outline of injury

Athletes involved in throwing sports are vulnerable to this condition, which is a result of severe stress to the elbow. The baseball pitch is a common source of thrower's elbow, as well as tennis, volleyball, javelin throwing, and cricket. Compression of the outer structures of the elbow combined with tension to the inner structures, over time, can cause painful stretching of ligaments as well as bone spurs and chips.

Anatomy and physiology

Although the elbow may be generally considered a hinge joint, it actually encompasses three articulations – the humero-ulnar, the humero-radial, and the proximal radio-ulnar joints. The three bones of the arm, the *humerus, radius* and *ulna*, help to form these joints. A forceful throwing motion can damage these bones, as well as the associated muscles, tendons, and ligaments of the elbow. Throwing activity results in a compression of structures on the lateral or outside of the elbow, while simultaneously stretching structures on the medial or inside of the elbow. Lateral compression can cause tiny fractures in the bones of the elbow, leading to bone spurs and chips. Medial stretching can cause a painful and debilitating strain to ligaments.

Cause of injury

Repetitive strain from throwing activity. Direct injury to the elbow. Improper athletic technique.

Signs and symptoms

Pain over both sides of the elbow. Weakness, stiffness or numbness of the elbow. Restricted mobility of the forearm due to elbow injury.

Complications if left unattended

Thrower's elbow eventually restricts movement in the arm and causes ongoing pain and inflammation. Bone spurs and chips, calcium formation, and the production of scar tissue are all symptomatic of this injury over time, if left unattended. Without proper treatment and rehabilitation, pressure on nerves and muscles due to such inflammation can restrict blood flow and pinch nerves used to control forearm muscles.

Immediate treatment

Avoidance of the activities causing repetitive stress to the elbow. R.I.C.E.R. regimen for 48–72 hours following injury. Use of anti-inflammatory drugs and analgesics.

Rehabilitation and prevention

Proper warm-up in order to prepare muscles and tendons for throwing activities is an essential preventive measure. Stretching exercises to maintain suppleness and flexibility of tendons should be an ongoing part of athletic preparation. Bracing and strapping the arm prior to throwing activity may also help to prevent thrower's elbow. Attention to proper equipment and technique is critical. Following a period of recovery from injury, exercises directed at regaining flexibility, endurance, and power should be undertaken.

Long-term prognosis

With proper rehabilitation, those suffering from thrower's elbow can generally expect a full recovery, though allowing the problem to worsen can lead to permanent, potentially career-ending restrictions of movement for athletes.

Brief outline of injury

Elbow bursitis, also known as *olecranon bursitis*, is caused by inflammation of small, fluid-filled sacs known as *bursae*. The function of a bursa is to provide a gliding surface that lubricates and reduces friction between various tissues in the body. Bursae tend to be located adjacent to tendons of major joints, including the shoulders, hips, knees, and elbows. Elbow bursitis occurs when the bursa below the tip of the elbow becomes inflamed from leaning on it too much or is injured through direct trauma.

Anatomy and physiology

The bony prominence at the tip of the elbow is known as the *olecranon process*. It is formed at the proximal aspect of the ulna. The fluid-filled sac located atop the olecranon process is the *olecranon bursa*, which is the largest bursa in the elbow region, and provides lubrication to underlying bone. Bursae are typically not visible unless bursitis has caused them to swell and become apparent. *Non-inflammatory bursitis* usually results from repeated trauma, such as leaning on the elbows, while *inflammatory bursitis* is the result of infection or an underlying inflammatory medical condition, e.g. rheumatism.

Cause of injury

A hard blow to the tip of the elbow, causing the bursa to swell with excess fluid. Leaning on the elbow tip for extended periods. An injury that breaks the skin, causing infection of the bursa.

Signs and symptoms

Pain in the elbow region at rest and during exercise. A rapid and painful swelling on the back of the elbow (red and warm, if infected). Swelling may stem from bleeding or seepage of fluid into the bursal sac. Reduced mobility in the elbow.

Complications if left unattended

In addition to continued pain, discomfort, and loss of elbow mobility, untreated bursitis can lead to more serious complications, especially when infection is present. In such cases, the fluid of the bursa can turn to pus, and the infection can intensify and spread in a condition known as *septic bursitis*, requiring aggressive medical treatment (including antibiotics and occasionally, a *bursectomy*—surgical removal of the infected bursa).

Immediate treatment

Rest the afflicted elbow, avoiding all unnecessary pressure. Ice compresses, anti-inflammatory medication, and analgesics.

Rehabilitation and prevention

The swollen bursa of the elbow may require aspiration by needle to drain fluid and reduce swelling. Cortisone injections may also be given, which can help prevent re-accumulation of fluid. Barring serious infection, these steps are generally sufficient to treat elbow bursitis. Protecting the elbow during athletics with bracing or padding, and avoiding excessive leaning on the point of the elbow can help prevent the injury.

Long-term prognosis

Long-term outlook for elbow bursitis is generally good, depending on the severity and nature of the injury. Most patients can expect full recovery, though complications can arise if infection is present, particularly if the condition is not given prompt medical attention.

Chapter

9

Sports Injuries of the Shoulder and Upper Arm

Acute

040: Fracture (Collar Bone, Humerus)

041: Dislocation of the Shoulder

042: Shoulder Subluxation

043: Acromioclavicular Separation

044: Sternoclavicular Separation

045: Biceps Brachii Tendon Rupture

046: Biceps Brachii Bruise

047: Muscle Strain (Biceps Brachii, Chest)

Chronic

048: Impingement Syndrome

049: Rotator Cuff Tendinitis

050: Shoulder Bursitis

051: Bicipital Tendinitis

052: Pectoral Muscle Insertion Inflammation

053: Frozen Shoulder (Adhesive Capsulitis)

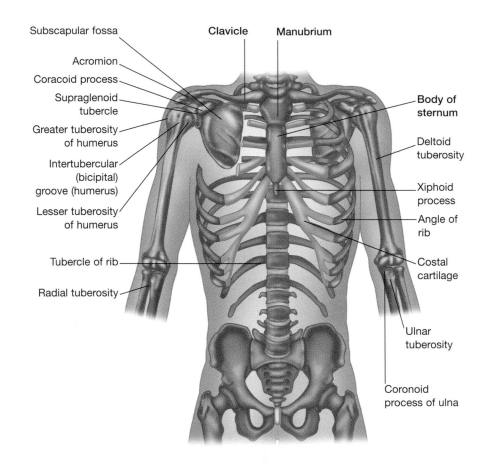

Subscapular fossa

Clavicle   Manubrium

Acromion

Coracoid process

Supraglenoid tubercle

Body of sternum

Greater tuberosity of humerus

Deltoid tuberosity

Intertubercular (bicipital) groove (humerus)

Xiphoid process

Angle of rib

Lesser tuberosity of humerus

Tubercle of rib

Costal cartilage

Radial tuberosity

Ulnar tuberosity

Coronoid process of ulna

Figure 9.1: Rib cage, pectoral girdle, upper arm (anterior view, the upper right anterior rib cage is removed).

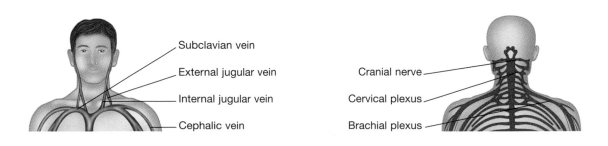

Subclavian vein

External jugular vein

Internal jugular vein

Cephalic vein

Cranial nerve

Cervical plexus

Brachial plexus

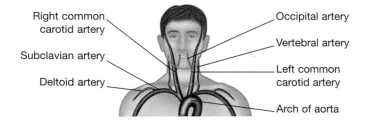

Right common carotid artery

Occipital artery

Vertebral artery

Subclavian artery

Deltoid artery

Left common carotid artery

Arch of aorta

040: FRACTURE (COLLAR BONE, HUMERUS)

Rehabilitation exercises

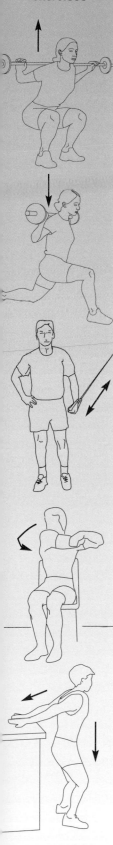

Brief outline of injury

Fractures of the shoulder usually involve a break in either the clavicle (collar bone) or the neck of the humerus (arm bone), or both. Impact injuries involving a sudden blow to the shoulder or a fall are usually responsible. Contact sports including football and rugby can result in shoulder fractures following a violent collision of two players.

Anatomy and physiology

The *clavicle* (collar bone) is a slender, doubly curved bone that attaches to the *manubrium* of the sternum medially (the sternoclavicular joint) and to the *acromion* of the scapula laterally (the acromioclavicular joint). The clavicle protects the underlying brachial plexus, pleural cap, and great vessels of the upper extremity. Clavicle fractures are common, often resulting from a fall on the lateral shoulder or on an outstretched arm. The *humerus* (arm bone) is the longest and largest bone of the upper limb. It articulates proximally with the scapula (at the *glenoid fossa*). Fractures to the humerus are generally the result of a fall on an outstretched arm.

Cause of injury

Fall on an outstretched arm. Sudden blow to the clavicle. Collision of two athletes in sports, e.g. football.

Signs and symptoms

Severe pain. Redness and bruising around the site of the injury. Inability to raise the arm.

Complications if left unattended

Complications are uncommon, although pneumothorax, haemothorax, and injuries to the brachial plexus or subclavian vessels are possible, requiring medical intervention. Chronic pain due to osteoarthritis may result should the injury be given insufficient time to heal.

Immediate treatment

Ice and analgesics for pain. Immobilization of the injured arm with a sling.

Rehabilitation and prevention

Bones of the clavicle and humerus must first be realigned following fracture, so that proper healing may ensue. Healing occurs while the clavicle and arm bones are held in place with a strap or sling. After healing, physical therapy, including range of motion and strengthening exercises should be undertaken to restore full movement and flexibility.

Long-term prognosis

Most shoulder fractures are successfully treated without resort to surgery, although this is occasionally required for fractures of the clavicle. For less severe fractures, full recovery and restoration of mobility may be expected. In the case of more severe fractures and particularly in older patients, some loss of motion and the possibility of osteoarthritis exist.

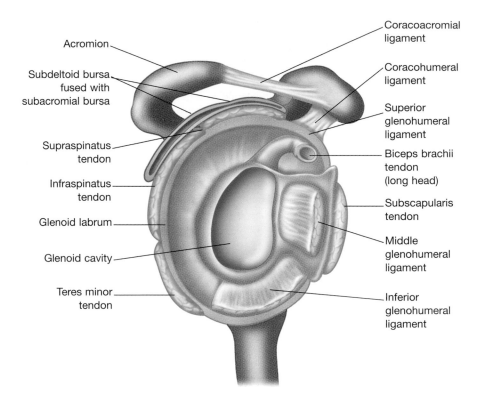

Acromion

Subdeltoid bursa fused with subacromial bursa

Supraspinatus tendon

Infraspinatus tendon

Glenoid labrum

Glenoid cavity

Teres minor tendon

Coracoacromial ligament

Coracohumeral ligament

Superior glenohumeral ligament

Biceps brachii tendon (long head)

Subscapularis tendon

Middle glenohumeral ligament

Inferior glenohumeral ligament

Figure 9.2: The shoulder joint (right arm, lateral view).

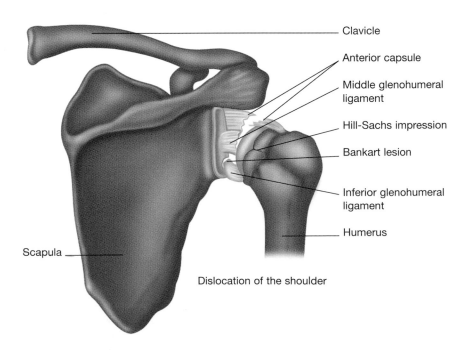

Clavicle

Anterior capsule

Middle glenohumeral ligament

Hill-Sachs impression

Bankart lesion

Inferior glenohumeral ligament

Humerus

Scapula

Dislocation of the shoulder

Rehabilitation exercises

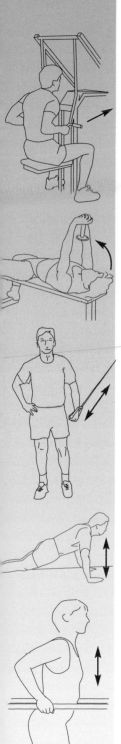

Brief outline of injury

Dislocation of the shoulder may occur when an athlete falls on an outstretched hand or during abduction and external rotation of the shoulder. Significant force is required to dislocate a shoulder, unless the athlete is experiencing re-injury. A shoulder dislocation occurs when the upper portion of the arm bone (humerus) pulls free of the socket of the shoulder-blade or scapula.

Anatomy and physiology

While several types of shoulder dislocation exist, the most common is *anterior dislocation*, which represents ninety-five percent of all cases. In this dislocation injury, the structures responsible for stabilizing the anterior shoulder, including the *anterior capsule* and the *inferior glenohumeral ligament*, are torn free from the bone. A compression fracture of the posteromedial humeral head is known as a *Hill-Sachs lesion*. More commonly, avulsion of the anterior glenoid labrum can occur, which is known as a *Bankart lesion*. Both often occur as a result of anterior dislocation of the shoulder.

Cause of injury

Violent contact with another athlete or solid object. A fall on an outstretched hand. Sudden, violent torsion of the shoulder.

Signs and symptoms

Severe pain in the shoulder. Arm held away from the body at the side, with the forearm turned outward. Irregular contour of the deltoid muscles.

Complications if left unattended

Dislocation of the shoulder causes tearing of the shoulder ligaments, resulting in the shoulder joint becoming less stable. This results in the shoulder capsule being considerably more prone to successive dislocations during athletics. Immobilization of the shoulder during the healing phase does not fully prevent such re-injury, which may require surgical intervention, since the immobilized ligament often fails to heal in the proper position.

Immediate treatment

Realignment or *reduction* of the dislocated joint. Immobilization and analgesics for pain.

Rehabilitation and prevention

Most initial shoulder dislocations are treated without resort to surgery, although subsequent dislocations may require surgical care, and many athletes suffer a range of disabilities following dislocation. An alternative to surgical treatment—*prolotherapy*—involves injections directed at the anterior shoulder capsule and the insertions of the middle and inferior glenohumeral ligaments. This may offer better relief from pain, restoration of mobility, and a speedier return to athletic activity. Further, the technique avoids the formation of scar tissue common after surgery.

Long-term prognosis

A large percentage of athletes may be unable to continue sports following a shoulder dislocation without subsequent injuries or the need for surgical treatment. Furthermore, athletes who undergo surgery following shoulder dislocation are often unable to perform at their former level. The alternative method of prolotherapy may offer relief and more effective healing.

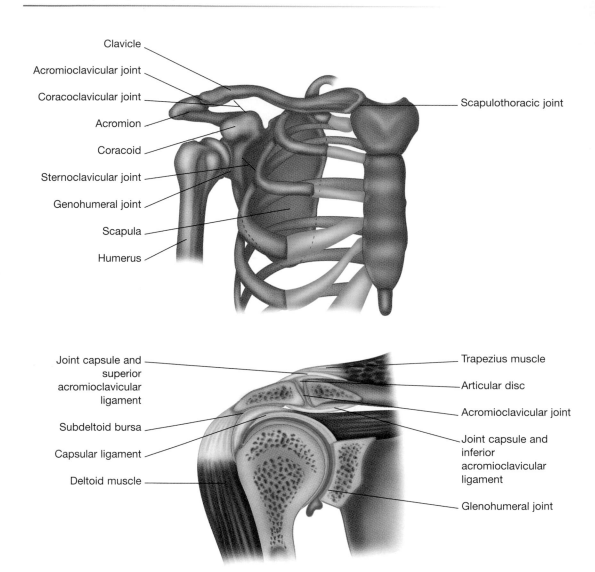

Clavicle

Acromioclavicular joint

Coracoclavicular joint

Acromion

Coracoid

Sternoclavicular joint

Genohumeral joint

Scapula

Humerus

Scapulothoracic joint

Joint capsule and superior acromioclavicular ligament

Subdeltoid bursa

Capsular ligament

Deltoid muscle

Trapezius muscle

Articular disc

Acromioclavicular joint

Joint capsule and inferior acromioclavicular ligament

Glenohumeral joint

Figure 9.3: The five joints of the shoulder region; the sternoclavicular (SC) joint, acromioclavicular (AC) joint, coracoclavicular joint, glenohumeral joint, and the scapulothoracic joint.

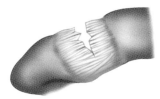

Separation

Rehabilitation exercises

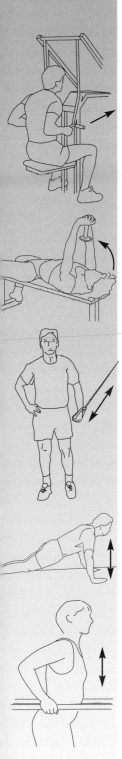

Brief outline of injury

The shoulder complex enables extreme mobility due to its anatomical structure, but provides little stability. Shoulder subluxation is a partial dislocation of the ball-and-socket joint of the shoulder. A group of ligaments securely hold the humerus (upper arm bone) in the socket of the shoulder-blade or scapula. Should these ligaments be torn, subluxation may result, in which the ball of the humerus slips partially out of the shoulder socket.

Anatomy and physiology

The shoulder region is actually composed of five joints: the sternoclavicular (SC) joint, the acromioclavicular (AC) joint, the coracoclavicular joint, the glenohumeral joint, and the scapulothoracic joint, where the shoulder-blade glides on the chest wall. The articulation referred to specifically as the *shoulder joint* is the glenohumeral joint, whereas the other articulations are joints of the *shoulder girdle*. The structure of the shoulder permits a wide arrange of motion, allowing the positioning of the arm and hand. Instability in the shoulder joint complex, particularly following dislocation, can result in subluxation.

Cause of injury

A direct blow to the shoulder. A fall onto an outstretched arm. Strenuously forcing the arm into an awkward position.

Signs and symptoms

Sensation of the shoulder going in and out of joint. Looseness of the shoulder joint. Pain, weakness, or numbness in the shoulder or arm.

Complications if left unattended

Untreated subluxation can cause wear, and ultimately damage the internal structures of the shoulder, sometimes requiring surgery. Loss of mobility, ongoing pain, and osteoarthritic complications may result from untreated subluxation.

Immediate treatment

R.I.C.E.R. regimen to reduce inflammation and treat pain. Anti-inflammatory medicines and analgesics for pain, e.g. *Ibuprofen*.

Rehabilitation and prevention

Following immobilization and healing, strengthening exercises should be undertaken. Recovery depends on factors including the athlete's age, health, history of previous injury, and severity of subluxation. If the shoulder subluxes frequently during activity, significant physical rehabilitation will be needed and possibly invasive surgery.

Long-term prognosis

Normal sports activity may be resumed once a full range of motion without subluxation has been achieved. Prognosis is dependent on the severity of the subluxation and the athlete's particular history. Subluxation is often due to previous shoulder injury and returning to athletics before full recovery can lead to further and worsening subluxation.

Brief outline of injury

Acromioclavicular separation is a separation of the ligaments that connect the clavicle (collar bone) to the shoulder bones (known as the *acromion process*). Acromioclavicular (AC) joint injuries generally occur in the course of upper-extremity strength training, various throwing sports, and collision sports (particularly, football and hockey). The injury is common among athletes in their 30's and 40's.

Anatomy and physiology

The arm is linked to the axial skeleton by means of the acromioclavicular joint, which connects the lateral end of the clavicle, and the medial border of the acromion of the scapula. A fibrocartilage articular disc partially divides the articular cavity, and absorbs forces and compression in the acromioclavicular joint. The acromioclavicular joint is stabilized by the anterior deltoid muscle, the trapezius muscle arising from the acromion, and additionally, by stabilizing ligaments.

Cause of injury

Fall onto the point of the shoulder. Fall onto an outstretched hand. Direct blow to the shoulder.

Signs and symptoms

Pain, tenderness, and swelling at the AC joint. Deformity of the injured joint. Pain or discomfort during cross-body adduction (turning the injured arm inward toward the opposite shoulder).

Complications if left unattended

Degenerative joint abnormalities, chronic pain and stiffness and limitations in mobility requiring surgery are possible, should the condition not be given prompt medical attention and allowed proper healing time.

Immediate treatment

Immobilization of the injured arm with a sling. Ice packs, rest, and the use of anti-inflammatory medication and analgesics for pain.

Rehabilitation and prevention

AC separations of a less severe nature are successfully treated without surgery, though a thorough healing period of 6–8 weeks is generally required, following which, range-of-motion exercises should be used to avoid stiffness. Exercises directed at maintaining strength and stability of the shoulder and upper back muscles may help prevent the injury, and use of padding around the AC joint, particularly during contact sports, may help avoid re-injury.

Long-term prognosis

Given adequate healing time and rehabilitation, most AC separations are resolved without surgery. Should surgery be required, risks of infection and continued pain exist, and recovery time for the athlete is lengthened.

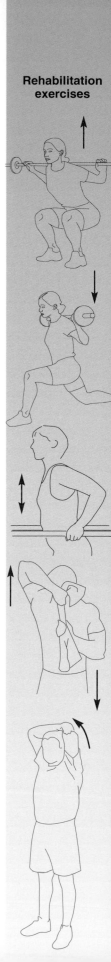

Rehabilitation exercises

**Rehabilitation
exercises**

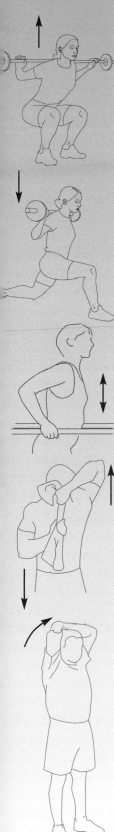

Brief outline of injury

Sternoclavicular separation occurs when a ligament connecting the collar bone or clavicle to the breastbone or sternum is torn. Rotation at the joint is affected by this injury, which may occur during contact sports when the shoulder forcefully strikes the ground or is landed upon by another player. The separation may occur anteriorly or posteriorly (in front of or behind the breastbone).

Anatomy and physiology

The sternoclavicular (SC) joint is functionally a ball-and-socket joint, but unlike most articular surfaces, the articular cartilage is fibrocartilage rather than hyaline cartilage. The SC joint is surrounded by a joint capsule, thickened anteriorly and posteriorly by: the posterior sternoclavicular ligament, the anterior sternoclavicular ligament, the costoclavicular ligament, and the interclavicular ligament. The sternoclavicular joint is strong and generally resistant to dislocation, and has a wide range of movement.

Cause of injury

Direct blow to the sternum. Fall onto the shoulder or outstretched hands. Shoulder striking the ground, or another athlete landing on top of the shoulder.

Signs and symptoms

Pain, swelling, and tenderness over the sternoclavicular joint. Abnormal movement between the breastbone and the collar bone. Possible displacement of the collar bone in front of or behind the breastbone.

Complications if left unattended

Untreated sternoclavicular separation can lead to loss of motion and ongoing pain, stiffness, and weakness. Furthermore, in cases where the collar bone is forced behind the breastbone, a risk exists for damage to the underlying blood vessels in the chest or the heart, requiring surgical intervention.

Immediate treatment

Reduction of the joint where needed, and immobilization with a sling. R.I.C.E.R. to reduce swelling, trauma, and pain.

Rehabilitation and prevention

As the injury is generally caused in a sports accident, prevention is usually not possible. In the case of anterior injury to the sternoclavicular joint (the most common), the condition is generally resolved without permanent complication, following adequate healing time. In more severe cases, surgery may be required. Range of motion exercises should help restore movement and rotational ability.

Long-term prognosis

With adequate time for healing, the injured athlete typically makes a full recovery. If the injury is serious (particularly in the case of posterior dislocation) instability of the joint may persist, in some cases requiring surgery.

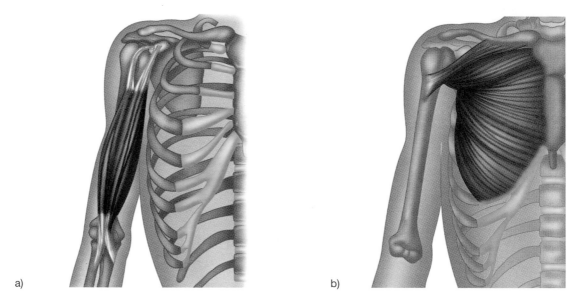

a) b)

Figure 9.4: a) The biceps brachii and, b) pectoralis major muscles.

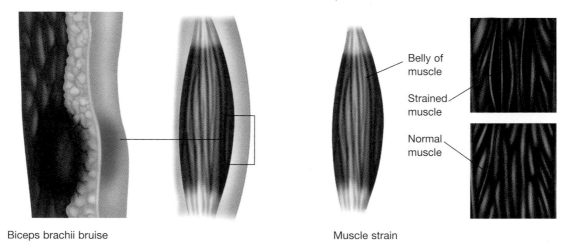

Biceps brachii bruise

Belly of
muscle

Strained
muscle

Normal
muscle

Muscle strain

045: BICEPS BRACHII TENDON RUPTURE

Rehabilitation exercises

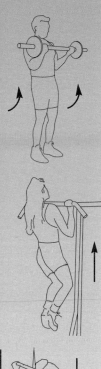

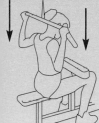

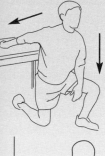

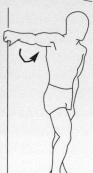

Brief outline of injury

Repetitive strain, particularly due to overlifting, can lead to irritation and microscopic tears in the biceps brachii tendon, which connects the biceps brachii muscle to the shoulder joint at the proximal end and the elbow at the muscle's distal end. A biceps brachii tendon rupture results from sudden trauma to the biceps brachii tendon causing its detachment from the bone. Injury at the proximal (shoulder) end of the tendon is most common. Biceps brachii tendon ruptures can occur from weight lifting or throwing sports, but are generally uncommon, particularly in young athletes.

Anatomy and physiology

The biceps brachii muscle is located on the front of the upper arm, and operates over three joints. Its function is to allow bending of the arm and to support loads placed on the arm. This muscle has two parts, known as the *long head* and *short head*, both connected to bone via the biceps brachii tendon. Rupture of the tendon prevents the muscle from pulling on the bone, thereby restricting movement. In older individuals, it is often the result of degenerative change in the tendon.

Cause of injury

Weakness due to tears in the rotator cuff. Throwing activities. Weightlifting.

Signs and symptoms

Bulge in the upper arm. Inability to turn the palm upward or downward. Sudden, sharp pain at the shoulder.

Complications if left unattended

Generally, little functional loss accompanies rupture of a proximal biceps brachii tendon, as two tendinous attachments occur at the shoulder, one compensating the other in most cases. For this reason, surgery is rarely required and complications are rare, though without proper healing, re-tearing and degeneration of the tendon are more likely.

Immediate treatment

Anti-inflammatory and analgesic medications such as *Ibuprofen* to reduce pain. R.I.C.E.R. regimen immediately following injury. Then heat to promote blood flow and healing.

Rehabilitation and prevention

Following rest and recovery of the tendon, flexibility and strengthening exercises should be undertaken to restore full mobility in the shoulder. Avoidance of sudden lifting beyond normal capacity and other sudden violence to the biceps brachii tendon as during throwing sports may help prevent the injury.

Long-term prognosis

Most biceps brachii tendon ruptures resolve themselves without medical intervention if given proper time for healing. In younger athletes with demanding training schedules, surgery may be contemplated to repair the rupture. Tears and ruptures to the distal end of the biceps brachii tendon at the elbow are more rare, but can be more severe, requiring surgery. However, in both cases the prospects for full recovery are excellent.

Brief outline of injury

Bruising to the biceps brachii can occur following tearing and/or rupture of the biceps brachii tendon, or trauma to the muscle. The biceps brachii tendon attaches the biceps brachii muscle to bone in the shoulder region. Overstrain from weight training can cause tears and bruising, which may also result from throwing sports or following direct trauma to the shoulder during a fall or collision with another athlete.

Anatomy and physiology

The biceps brachii muscle is located on the front of the upper arm, and operates over three joints. Its function is to allow bending of the arm and to support loads placed on the arm. This muscle has two parts, known as the *long head* and *short head*, both connected to bone via the biceps brachii tendon. This muscle runs down the anterior or front side of the upper arm and allows motion of the forearm towards the shoulder (elbow flexion). The biceps brachii muscle also allows turning the hand face down or face up. This is known as *pronation* or *supination* of the forearm.

Cause of injury

Direct blow to the biceps brachii region of the upper arm. Biceps brachii rupture. Repetitive tearing of the biceps brachii muscle or tendon.

Signs and symptoms

Discolouration of the biceps brachii area. Aches or pain in the biceps brachii. Stiffness and limitations of movement in the affected arm and shoulder.

Complications if left unattended

Bruising of the biceps brachii generally resolves itself without treatment. Sports involving heavy use of the biceps brachii muscle including weight training and throwing sports, and contact activities with high risk to the biceps brachii should be avoided pending adequate time for healing.

Immediate treatment

R.I.C.E.R. regimen to reduce inflammation and treat pain. Immobilization with a sling to prevent excess movement.

Rehabilitation and prevention

Rest and avoidance of activities involving stress to the biceps brachii muscle and tendons during the healing phase are generally sufficient. Range of motion exercises and graded strength training should be undertaken to restore full power and resilience to the muscle. Stretching exercises performed before athletic activity may help prevent injury and associated bruising to the biceps brachii.

Long-term prognosis

Bruising to the biceps brachii is generally a minor condition that is self-correcting without resort to surgery, given adequate time for healing. No long-term deficit in strength or mobility is expected.

Rehabilitation exercises

**Rehabilitation
exercises**

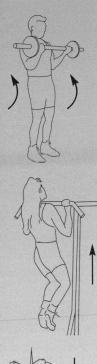

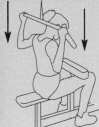

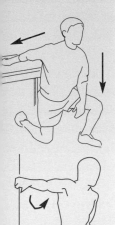

Brief outline of injury

Muscle strains are among the most common sports injuries and often result from the sudden extension of a joint beyond its normal range of function. This causes damage to muscle and other soft tissue. The chest muscles (pectoralis major and minor) join the biceps brachii muscle at the shoulder joint. Weight training, sudden, violent torsion of the shoulder during throwing sports, or a sudden force applied to the nexus of the pectorals and biceps brachii (as when warding off a check in hockey with the arm extended), can produce such injuries.

Anatomy and physiology

The biceps brachii muscle is located on the front of the upper arm, and operates over three joints. Its function is to allow bending of the arm and to support loads placed on the arm. This muscle has two parts, known as the *long head* and *short head*, both connected to bone via the biceps brachii tendon.

Along with the pectoralis minor, the large pectoralis major muscle forms the anterior wall of the axilla, and has its origin in the clavicle, sternum, and first six costal cartilages, inserting in the greater tubercle of the humerus bone. The muscle is used for flexion, adduction, and medial rotation. It joins the biceps brachii muscle, meeting at the shoulder joint.

Cause of injury

Sudden movement leading to a muscle tear. Large physical demand placed on the muscle. Warding off a check in hockey or tackle in football.

Signs and symptoms

Tenderness and pain over the affected muscle. Stiffness. Pain during muscle use.

Complications if left unattended

Muscle strains are usually self-limiting and repair themselves given proper time off from exertion and allowing time for healing. Insufficient recovery time however can lead to further tearing, increasing the risk of re-injury and lead to degenerative changes in the muscles over time.

Immediate treatment

R.I.C.E.R. regimen to reduce inflammation and treat pain. Analgesics for muscle pain combined with anti-inflammatory medication. Then heat to promote blood flow and healing.

Rehabilitation and prevention

Stretching exercises following healing can help restore full mobility in the affected area while strengthening exercises can help prevent re-injury. Stretching and warm-up, as well as attention to proper athletic technique (particularly in weight training) may help prevent this type of injury.

Long-term prognosis

Muscle strains involving the pectoral muscles of the chest and/or the biceps brachii are common and—given adequate time for proper healing—generally not a serious threat to the athlete, although severe or repeated muscle strains can cause chronic pain and lead to impairment of muscle function.

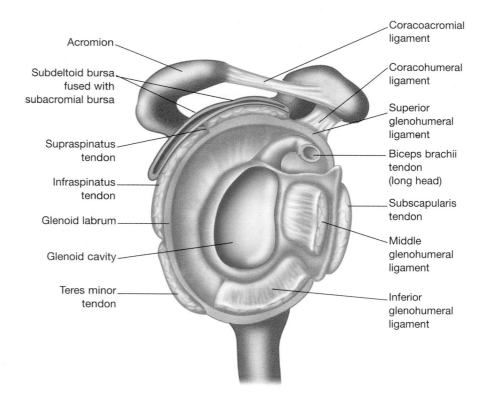

Coracoacromial ligament

Coracohumeral ligament

Superior glenohumeral ligament

Biceps brachii tendon (long head)

Subscapularis tendon

Middle glenohumeral ligament

Inferior glenohumeral ligament

Acromion

Subdeltoid bursa fused with subacromial bursa

Supraspinatus tendon

Infraspinatus tendon

Glenoid labrum

Glenoid cavity

Teres minor tendon

Figure 9.5: The shoulder joint, right arm, lateral view.

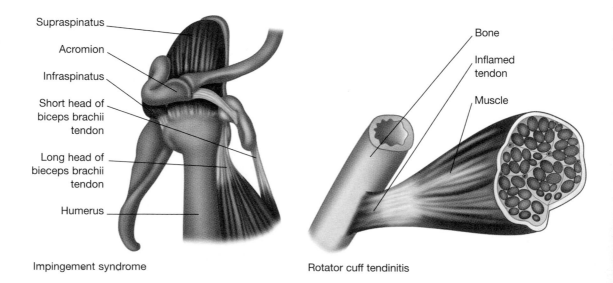

Supraspinatus

Acromion

Infraspinatus

Short head of biceps brachii tendon

Long head of biceps brachii tendon

Humerus

Impingement syndrome

Bone

Inflamed tendon

Muscle

Rotator cuff tendinitis

Rehabilitation exercises

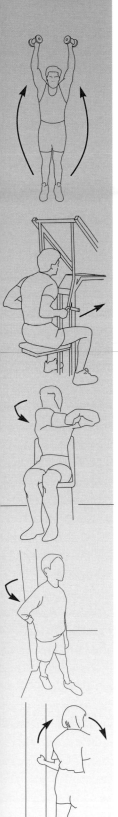

Brief outline of injury

Impingement syndrome is a chronic condition caused by repetitive overhead activity or throwing events that damage the glenoid labrum, long head of the biceps brachii, and the subacromial bursa. A narrowing of the space between the rotator cuff and the acromion results in shoulder pain and loss of movement, due to deficit in the affected rotator cuff, a group of muscles and tendons necessary to secure the arm to the shoulder joint. The rotator cuff permits free rotation of the arm.

Anatomy and physiology

The *rotator cuff* is composed of four muscles: *subscapularis, supraspinatus, infraspinatus,* and *teres minor*, as well as their musculo-tendinous attachments. The *subacromial bursa* (a fluid-filled sac), is the largest and most commonly injured bursa in the shoulder region, and provides the rotator cuff with lubrication to assist movement. The rotator cuff acts to stabilize the glenohumeral joint. Damage, including tears to the rotator cuff, can cause the humeral head to migrate during elevation of the arm, leading to impingement.

Cause of injury

Repeated overhead movements as in tennis, swimming, golf, and weight lifting. Irritation of the rotator cuff due to throwing sports including baseball. Underlying predisposition, including rheumatoid arthritis.

Signs and symptoms

Shoulder pain and difficulty raising the arm in the air. Pain during sleep when the injured arm is rolled on. Pain during rotational movements such as reaching into a back pocket.

Complications if left unattended

Increasing stiffness of the joint and further loss of motion may result should impingement be ignored. Rotator tendons may be torn, should athletic activity be undertaken prior to full recovery. Tendinitis and bursitis frequently develop with impingement as a pre-condition.

Immediate treatment

Rest, ice packs, and anti-inflammatory medication. Corticosteroid injections may be used under the acromion to reduce inflammation.

Rehabilitation and prevention

Following a period of healing, physical therapy will often be used to restore strength and range of motion in the affected rotator cuff. Avoiding or limiting repetitive motions that cause rotator cuff irritation may help prevent the injury. Strengthening exercises and lightweight training to strengthen the muscles of the rotator cuff are also useful preventive measures.

Long-term prognosis

Typically, the condition shows marked improvement within 6–12 weeks. In cases where recovery has not been achieved in 6–12 months, surgery may be recommended to release the ligaments. Surgery is usually followed by physical therapy, and some modification of athletic activity may be necessary to reduce the chances of relapse.

Brief outline of injury

Rotator cuff tendinitis results from the irritation and inflammation of the tendons of the shoulder in the area underlying the acromion. The condition is sometimes known as *pitcher's shoulder* though it is a common injury in all sports requiring overhead arm movements, including tennis, volleyball, swimming and weight lifting, in addition to baseball.

Anatomy and physiology

The shoulder (or *glenohumeral*) joint is a ball-and-socket structure formed by the top portion of the arm bone (humerus) associated with the scapula or shoulder-blade. The rotator cuff aligns the head of the humerus into the scapula. Occasionally, following repetitive use of the rotator cuff, the humerus can ride up to pinch the cuff and irritate the fluid-filled *subacromial bursa* that acts to cushion the rotator cuff and acromion / humerus.

Cause of injury

Inflammation of the tendons of the shoulder from tennis, baseball, swimming, etc. Irritation of the bursa of the rotator cuff from repetitive overhead arm motion. Pre-existing disposition including anatomical irregularity.

Signs and symptoms

Weakness or pain with overhead activities, brushing hair, reaching, etc. Popping or cracking sensation in the shoulder. Pain in the injured shoulder, particularly when lying on it.

Complications if left unattended

Rotator cuff tendinitis can worsen without attention as the tendons and bursa become increasingly inflamed. Motion becomes more limited and tendon tears can cause further, in some cases, chronic pain. Further, the acromion may react to prolonged irritation with the production of *bone spurs*, which contribute to further irritation.

Immediate treatment

Application of ice and use of anti-inflammatory medication. Discontinue all athletic and other activity causing rotator cuff pain. Then heat to promote blood flow and healing.

Rehabilitation and prevention

Following rest and healing of the injured shoulder, physical therapy should be undertaken to strengthen the muscles of the rotator cuff. Occasionally, steroid injections are required to reduce pain and inflammation. Moderation of rotator cuff use, adequate recovery time between athletic activities, and strength training can all help avoid the injury.

Long-term prognosis

Given proper rest as well as physical therapy and (where needed) steroidal injections, most athletes enjoy a full recovery from this injury. Should a serious tear of the rotator cuff tissue occur, surgery may be required, although a recovery to pre-injury levels of activity is usually expected.

Rehabilitation exercises

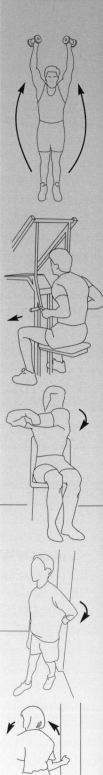

130

050: SHOULDER BURSITIS

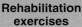

Rehabilitation exercises

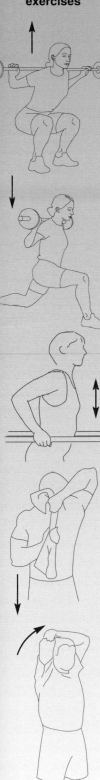

Brief outline of injury

Shoulder bursitis is not generally an isolated condition, but is usually associated with a rotator cuff tear, or impingement syndrome, and occurs when the region between the upper arm bone (*humerus*) and the tip of the shoulder (*acromion*) becomes inflamed. Tennis, baseball, and weight training are all prone to this injury.

Anatomy and physiology

Tendons of the rotator cuff act to rotate the upper humerus, raising the arm by pulling the humeral head down. At the same time, the deltoid muscle pulls the arm up. This process can lead to irritation due to pressure from the acromion process of the scapula and the coraco-acromial ligament. Such irritation can affect the bursae—fluid-filled sacs providing a cushion between the bones and the tendons—leading to inflammation and accumulation of excess fluid, further limiting the space available for tendon movement. The *subacromial bursa* is the largest and most commonly injured bursa in the shoulder region.

Cause of injury

Overuse of the shoulder from throwing activities, tennis, swimming or baseball. Falling onto an outstretched arm. Infection of the bursa in the shoulder.

Signs and symptoms

Pain in the shoulder, particularly when raising the arm. Pain when turning over in bed on the injured shoulder. Loss of strength and limited motion of the shoulder.

Complications if left unattended

Failure to attend to shoulder bursitis generally results in a worsening of the condition, a further thickening of tendons and bursa(e) leading to increased inflammation and pain. The athlete runs the risk of developing a chronic condition, as well as a danger that the fluid in the bursa(e) becomes infected, a potentially serious situation, sometimes necessitating surgery.

Immediate treatment

Discontinue all activity causing inflammation of the shoulder. R.I.C.E.R. regimen to reduce inflammation and treat pain. Then heat to promote blood flow and healing.

Rehabilitation and prevention

The athlete should avoid pressure to the injured shoulder and inflamed bursa(e) during recovery as well as any activities likely to irritate the condition. Begin exercising the shoulder when instructed by a medical professional in order to restore strength and shoulder mobility. Warming-up and cooling-down exercises, with an emphasis on stretching, strength training and maintaining looseness in the shoulder can help prevent bursitis from developing.

Long-term prognosis

Shoulder bursitis tends to ease with proper healing and minor rehabilitation, and a full recovery to athletic activity can usually be expected, particularly if no infection of the bursa is detected. In some cases, aspiration of bursa fluid by needle is recommended to reduce inflammation and ensure no infection is present.

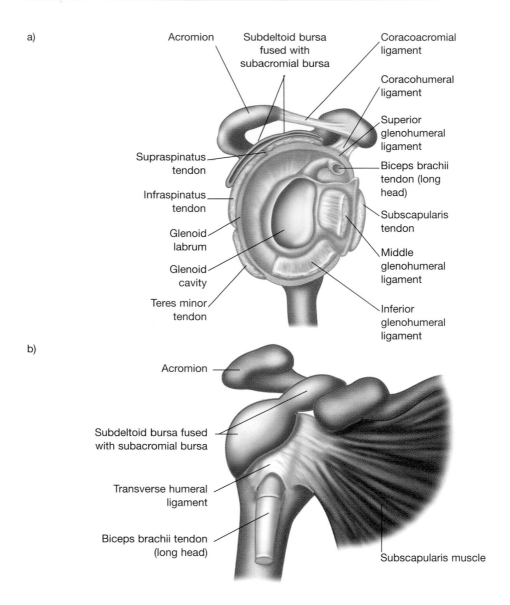

a)

Acromion

Subdeltoid bursa fused with subacromial bursa

Coracoacromial ligament

Coracohumeral ligament

Superior glenohumeral ligament

Supraspinatus tendon

Biceps brachii tendon (long head)

Infraspinatus tendon

Subscapularis tendon

Glenoid labrum

Middle glenohumeral ligament

Glenoid cavity

Teres minor tendon

Inferior glenohumeral ligament

b)

Acromion

Subdeltoid bursa fused with subacromial bursa

Transverse humeral ligament

Biceps brachii tendon (long head)

Subscapularis muscle

Figure 9.6: a) The shoulder joint; right arm, lateral view, b) right arm, anterior view (cut).

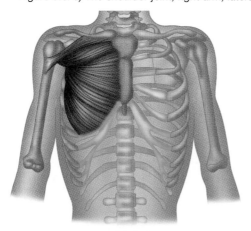

Figure 9.7: The pectoralis major muscle.

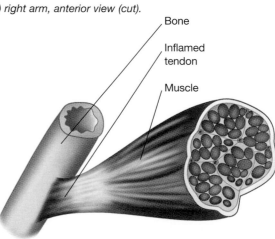

Bone

Inflamed tendon

Muscle

Bicipital tendinitis

051: BICIPITAL TENDINITIS

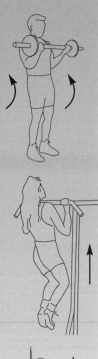

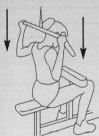

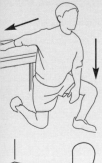

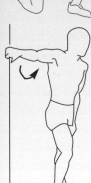

Brief outline of injury

Bicipital tendinitis results from irritation and inflammation to the biceps brachii tendon, which lies on the front of the shoulder and allows bending of the elbow and supination of the forearm. Overuse can lead to inflammation and is a common affliction in golfers, weight lifters, rowers, and those engaged in throwing sports.

Anatomy and physiology

Tendons are tough, resilient bands of fibrous tissue, connecting muscle to the bone. Irritation of the tendon due to overuse occurs as it passes back and forth in the intertubercular (bicipital) groove of the humerus, and can cause inflammation of the tendons (known as *tendinitis*) as well as the tendon sheaths or *paratenons*. The musculo-tendinous junction of the biceps brachii is highly susceptible to injuries brought on by overuse, particularly following repetitive lifting activities.

Cause of injury

Poor technique, particularly in weight lifting. Sudden increase in duration or intensity of training. Impingement syndrome.

Signs and symptoms

Pain over the bicipital groove when the tendon is passively stretched, and during resisted supination and elbow flexion. Pain and tenderness along the tendon length. Stiffness following exercise.

Complications if left unattended

Bicipital tendinitis, left without care and treatment, generally worsens as the biceps brachii tendon becomes increasingly irritated and inflamed. Movement and the ability to perform athletically without pain will be further hampered. Exercising without adequate healing and rehabilitation can lead to tearing of the tendon and tendon degeneration over time.

Immediate treatment

R.I.C.E.R. regimen to relieve painful inflammation. Anti-inflammatory and analgesic medication. Then heat to promote blood flow and healing.

Rehabilitation and prevention

The condition is self-limiting given rest and minimal medical attention. Following full recovery, exercises directed at improving flexibility, proprioception, and strength may be undertaken. Thorough warming-up and stretching exercises and a steady athletic regimen that avoids sudden, unprepared increases in activity can help avoid this injury, as can attention to proper sports technique.

Long-term prognosis

A full return to athletic activity may generally be expected, given adequate time for tendon recovery and reduction of inflammation. However, the injury is frequently recurrent. Surgery is generally not required. Injections of steroid or cortisone are sometimes used to reduce pain, though they must be applied cautiously, as they increase the risk of weakening or rupture of the tendon.

052: PECTORAL MUSCLE INSERTION INFLAMMATION

Brief outline of injury

The pectoralis major or pectoral muscle is used in many sports when the arms act to push away a weight (as during weight lifting) or another athlete (during various contact sports). Repetitive activity, particularly bench pressing, can cause irritation to the muscle or tendon's insertion point, leading to discomfort and loss of mobility.

Anatomy and physiology

The large pectoralis major muscle forms the anterior wall of the axilla, and has its origin in the clavicle, sternum, and first six costal cartilages, inserting in the greater tubercle of the humerus bone. The muscle adducts and medially rotates the humerus. The *clavicular portion* flexes and medially rotates the shoulder joint, and horizontally adducts the humerus towards the opposite shoulder. The *sternocostal portion* obliquely adducts the humerus towards the opposite hip. It is one of the main climbing muscles, pulling the body up to the fixed arm.

Cause of injury

Excessive load on the pectoralis major muscle, especially when bench-pressing. Excessive force against the pectoral from pushing activities in contact sports. A fall on to one or both outstretched arms.

Signs and symptoms

Pain and weakness in the shoulder. Difficulty raising the arm. Pain or stiffness during lifting.

Complications if left unattended

Irritation of the pectoral muscle insertion will become further aggravated if it is neglected. Tears in the muscle or tendon can develop, leading to increased pain and weakness and the danger of long-term degeneration of muscle and tendon. Should tearing at the insertion point become serious, surgery may be required to repair it.

Immediate treatment

Immediate cessation to athletic activity causing irritation. R.I.C.E.R. regimen to reduce inflammation and treat pain. Then heat to promote blood flow and healing.

Rehabilitation and prevention

Thorough healing time must be allowed for the pectoral muscle and associated tendons. Strength training of the pectorals through weights and graded calisthenics will generally help restore the athlete to prior condition, providing that no serious tearing of the muscle has resulted. Attention to proper weight training technique and a gradual, rather than sudden increase in stress on the pectoral muscle, can help prevent this injury.

Long-term prognosis

Given proper care and healing time, combined with gradual strength training of the pectoral muscles and complex of shoulder muscles, the athlete may generally expect a full return to normal activity.

Rehabilitation exercises

053: FROZEN SHOULDER (ADHESIVE CAPSULITIS)

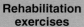
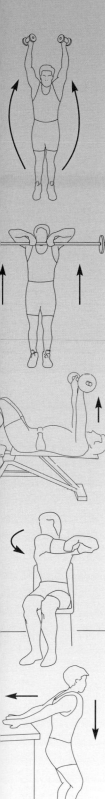

Brief outline of injury

Frozen shoulder or *adhesive capsulitis* causes severe restriction of shoulder movement due to pain. The condition results from abnormal bands of tissue that form between joints, thereby restricting their motion and producing pain. *Synovial fluid*—which usually serves to lubricate the space between the capsule and ball of the humerus in the shoulder, allowing smooth motion—is often lacking in this condition. It is more common in females.

Anatomy and physiology

Frozen shoulder involves injury and accompanying loss of movement in the shoulder or glenohumeral joint. The joint consists of a ball (formed by the humeral head) and socket (the glenoid cavity). While the glenohumeral joint is normally one of the body's most mobile joints, it is inherently unstable due to the glenoid cavity being only approximately one-third the size of the humeral head, (although it is slightly deepened by a rim of fibrocartilage called the *glenoid labrum*). The joint capsule appears to be a major source of movement limitation in this condition. Adhesions of scar tissue forming in joint spaces can restrict movement, causing the shoulder to freeze up, with severely limited range of motion.

Cause of injury

Scar tissue formation following shoulder injury. Formation of adhesions following shoulder surgery. Repeated tearing of soft tissue surrounding the glenohumeral joint.

Signs and symptoms

Dull, aching pain in the shoulder region, often worsening at night. Restricted movement of the shoulder. Pain and ache when lifting the affected arm.

Complications if left unattended

Frozen shoulder has a tendency to worsen over time without adequate treatment and proper recovery period. Attempted athletic activity, involving the affected shoulder, will likely lead to further adhesions of the joint, with further pain and restrictions of movement. Production of scar tissue may eventually require surgical removal.

Immediate treatment

Application of moist heat to the shoulder to loosen the affected joint. Muscle relaxants to relax shoulder muscles and arm.

Rehabilitation and prevention

Moist heat should be accompanied by stretching exercises to gradually restore mobility. Heat therapy should be combined with doctor-supervised physical therapy. Moving the shoulder through the full range of motion several times daily, as well as strength training exercises, may help avoid frozen shoulder. Injuries to the shoulder should be given prompt medical attention to avoid formation of scar tissue, where possible.

Long-term prognosis

The length of recovery time following frozen shoulder varies depending on the underlying cause as well as the age and health of the athlete, and the history of shoulder injury. If the condition fails to improve after 4–6 months, surgery may be required. Some lasting discomfort and impairment of movement is common with this injury.

Chapter

10

Sports Injuries of the
Back and Spine

Acute

054: Muscle Strain of the Back

055: Ligament Sprain of the Back

056: Thoracic Contusion

Chronic

057: Slipped Disc (Herniated or Ruptured)

058: Bulging Disc

059: Stress Fracture of the Vertebra

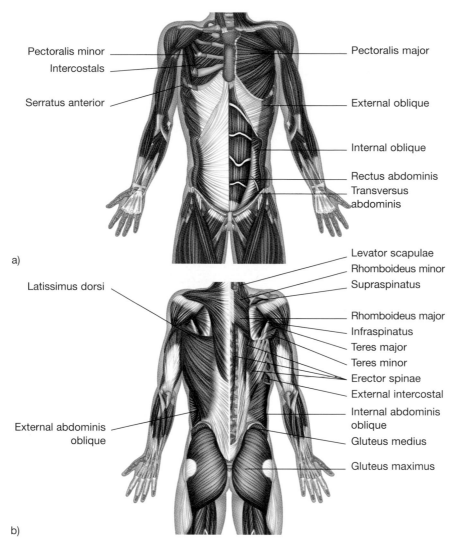

Pectoralis minor

Intercostals

Serratus anterior

Pectoralis major

External oblique

Internal oblique

Rectus abdominis

Transversus abdominis

a)

Levator scapulae

Rhomboideus minor

Supraspinatus

Latissimus dorsi

Rhomboideus major

Infraspinatus

Teres major

Teres minor

Erector spinae

External intercostal

Internal abdominis oblique

External abdominis oblique

Gluteus medius

Gluteus maximus

b)

Figure 10.1: Muscles of the thoracic region, a) anterior view, b) posterior view.

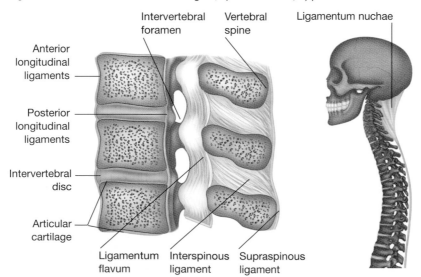

Intervertebral foramen

Vertebral spine

Ligamentum nuchae

Anterior longitudinal ligaments

Posterior longitudinal ligaments

Intervertebral disc

Articular cartilage

Ligamentum flavum

Interspinous ligament

Supraspinous ligament

Figure 10.2: Sagittal section of vertebrae.

Strained muscle

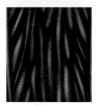

Normal muscle

Muscle strain

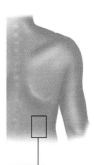

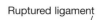

Thoracic contusion

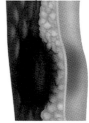

Ruptured ligament

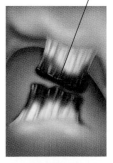

Ligament sprain of the back

Rehabilitation exercises

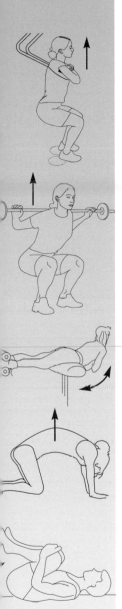

Brief outline of injury

Back strain occurs from a stretching injury to the muscles or tendons of the back. It is a common sports injury that can result from lifting, sudden movement, or a fall, collision with another athlete, or any activity in which the muscles of the back are engaged. Back strain often affects the lower back or lumbar region and the pain associated with this injury ranges from moderate to severe.

Anatomy and physiology

Three types of muscles occur in the back: *extensors* (including gluteal muscles), *flexors* (including the abdominal muscles and iliopsoas muscles) and *obliques* or *rotators* (side muscles). Back strain frequently involves the lower back or lumbar spine, which is composed of five spinal bones or vertebrae and the sacrum, which provide support and protection of the spinal cord.

Cause of injury

Sudden strain on the back muscles from lifting. Abrupt movement involving muscles of the back. Repetitive stress to the back muscles.

Signs and symptoms

Pain, stiffness, and loss of movement in the back. Rigidity in the back. Tingling and sensitivity.

Complications if left unattended

Muscle strains in the back usually resolve themselves with proper rest. Ignoring muscle strain however can lead to chronic back pain, stiffness and discomfort, with degeneration of the muscles and tendons. Muscle spasms accompanying inflammation can cause further pain, in some cases, severe.

Immediate treatment

Rest on a firm surface, lying on the back rather than the stomach. Ice pack, analgesic, and anti-inflammatory drugs.

Rehabilitation and prevention

After use of ice to reduce inflammation, heat therapy in modest amounts may help ease discomfort. Recovery times for muscle strain in the back vary widely depending on the severity of the strain, location, and overall health of the athlete. When the muscles have begun to heal, it is important that they receive moderate use, to avoid wasting and atrophy. Later, exercises to strengthen the back and restore mobility can help avoid recurrence of this injury.

Long-term prognosis

Muscle strains in the back, though sometimes quite painful, usually heal thoroughly with no residual loss of movement or pain, though some risk of re-injury exists, particularly if the strain was severe. Surgery is not required in cases of muscle strain, providing no severe tearing of tissue or tendon is involved.

SPORTS INJURIES OF THE BACK AND SPINE

Brief outline of injury

Sudden, irregular motion, repetitive stress or excessive load on the ligaments associated with the back can cause a sprain, or tearing of the ligaments. The resulting injury, which affects athletes in a broad variety of sports, produces pain and varying degrees of immobility.

Anatomy and physiology

Ligaments are resilient bands made up of fibrous tissue. They provide strong, flexible linkages between bones. A number of ligaments support the spine. The anterior and posterior longitudinal ligaments connect the vertebral bodies in the cervical, thoracic, and lumbar regions. The supraspinous ligament attaches to the spinous processes, and is enlarged in the cervical region, where it is known as the *ligamentum nuchae*. The *ligamenta flava* attach to, and extend between the ventral portions of the laminae of two adjacent vertebrae, from C2/C3 to L5/S1. The ligaments, muscles, and tendons work together to manage external forces to the spine during movement, particularly, bending motions and lifting.

Cause of injury

Lifting beyond normal capacity. Sudden torsion of the spine, including a fall during skiing or other sport. Unprepared movement involving the back.

Signs and symptoms

Pain and stiffness. Difficulty bending over and pain when straightening the back. Tenderness and inflammation of the back.

Complications if left unattended

A sprain to the ligaments will generally force the athlete to rest the injury and allow healing time due to pain and stiffness precluding normal activity. Should activity be continued before adequate healing, further tearing of the ligaments and lasting ligament injury may result. A mild ligament sprain can become acutely painful and incapacitating if ignored.

Immediate treatment

R.I.C.E.R. regimen immediately following injury. Non-steroidal anti-inflammatory drugs (NSAIDs).

Rehabilitation and prevention

In the case of mild to moderate ligament sprain, a few days rest should allow a return to most non-athletic daily activity. This should be undertaken to re-establish flexibility in the spine and avoid atrophy. Strengthening exercises for the back should not be undertaken until full recovery. Warm-ups and stretching prior to sports, proper posture and attention to proper technique can help avoid this injury.

Long-term prognosis

Less than 5% of back injuries require surgery, and surgery is rarely warranted for ligament sprain, although 6–8 weeks of recovery are often required, sometimes longer, should the sprain be serious. Failure to allow complete healing will increase the risk of re-injury.

Rehabilitation exercises

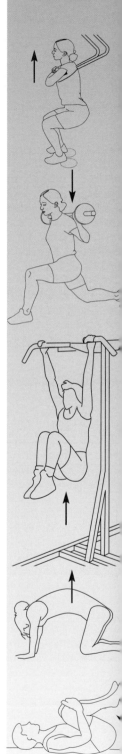

056: THORACIC CONTUSION

Rehabilitation exercises

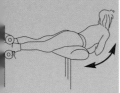

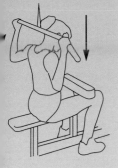

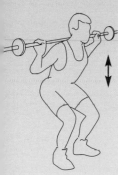

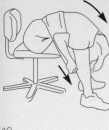

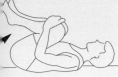

Brief outline of injury

A contusion is a closed wound to the body's soft tissue, resulting from a blow to muscle, tendon, or ligament. Contusion injuries cause bruising and often, discolouration, due to blood pooling around the site of trauma. Contusions of the back are possible in a variety of contact sports like football and hockey, due to violent force applied to the soft tissues, or as the result of a fall on the back.

Anatomy and physiology

Contusions involve trauma to the subcutaneous tissue. Because the musculature is well vascularized and the regional blood flow is usually high at the moment of impact, bleeding occurs from torn blood vessels into the skin and subcutaneous tissues, forming a bruise or *ecchymosis* (discolouration of an area of the skin). Capillaries are damaged due to blunt force, resulting in blood seeping into the surrounding tissue. While most contusions acquired in the course of sports activity are minor, some are symptomatic of serious injuries including fractures or internal bleeding.

Cause of injury

Overloading or overstretching muscles through a blow to the back from another athlete during contact sports. Blow from sports equipment, especially hockey and lacrosse. Hard fall on the back.

Signs and symptoms

Pain at injury site. Tenderness to the touch. Blue, purple, orange or yellow discolouration of the skin. Painful spasms and knot-like contractions (which act as a protective mechanism).

Complications if left unattended

Contusions may indicate more serious underlying conditions, including fracture, haematoma (blood in the muscle), or other internal bleeding, all of which should receive prompt medical attention. Minor contusions generally clear up in a matter of days without complication. More severe cases, however, may require 3–4 weeks to heal.

Immediate treatment

Rest, discontinue activity, and apply ice to reduce swelling. Anti-inflammatory medication and analgesics for pain, if needed. Activity modification.

Rehabilitation and prevention

Avoiding pressure or further trauma to the contusion site and application of ice are usually sufficient to speed recovery. As contusions result from blunt force accidents, they are generally not preventable, though proper conditioning and diet (including an abundance of vitamin C) may lessen the severity of contusion. Follow-up management may include application of superficial heat, ultrasound, massage, and appropriate stretching and resistance exercise.

Long-term prognosis

While contusions in the back can produce significant acute pain, they are faster to heal than muscle strains or ligament sprains. Severity of bruising depends on many factors, including muscle tension or relaxation at the time of injury. Pain will generally subside in hours or days and skin discolouration will abate as well. The athlete should enjoy a full return to activity, in more severe cases after about 4 weeks, without lasting deficit.

SPORTS INJURIES OF THE BACK AND SPINE

SPORTS INJURIES OF THE BACK AND SPINE

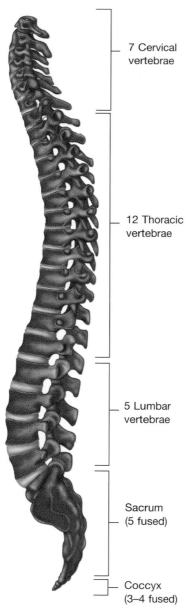

7 Cervical
vertebrae

12 Thoracic
vertebrae

5 Lumbar
vertebrae

Sacrum
(5 fused)

Coccyx
(3–4 fused)

Figure 10.3: The vertebral column, lateral view.

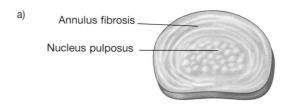

a)
Annulus fibrosis

Nucleus pulposus

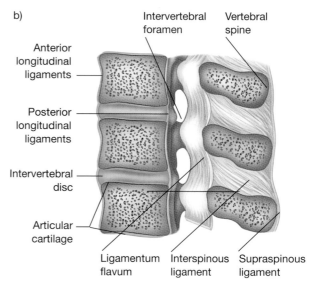

b)
Intervertebral foramen   Vertebral spine

Anterior longitudinal ligaments

Posterior longitudinal ligaments

Intervertebral disc

Articular cartilage

Ligamentum flavum   Interspinous ligament   Supraspinous ligament

*Figure 10.4: Vertebrae; a) sagittal section,
b) transverse section of intervertebral disc.*

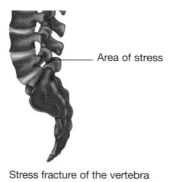

Area of stress

Stress fracture of the vertebra

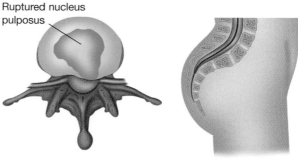

Ruptured nucleus pulposus

Slipped disc

057: SLIPPED DISC (HERNIATED OR RUPTURED)

Rehabilitation exercises

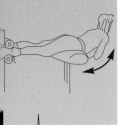

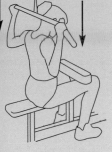

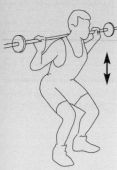

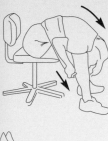

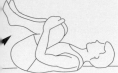

Brief outline of injury

A slipped disc (also known as *herniated, ruptured,* or *prolapsed disc*) results when the shock-absorbing pads or intervertebral discs filling the spaces between the bones of the spine, split or rupture. The discs contain a jelly-like substance that seeps out into the surrounding tissue, causing pressure and pain to the spinal cord or spinal nerves in the area of rupture. Slipped discs most frequently occur in the lower back although any disc of the spine is vulnerable to rupture.

Anatomy and physiology

The spine is made up of bones known as *vertebrae*, separated by fibrocartilaginous intervertebral discs. There is only slight movement between any two successive vertebrae, but there is considerable movement throughout the spinal column as a whole. The intervertebral discs are composed of a thick ring of fibrous cartilage, known as the *annulus fibrosis* which surrounds a jelly-like material known as the *nucleus pulposus*, and provide flexibility, cushioning, and protection to the spine. The *spinal canal* runs through the center of the vertebrae and discs and contains the spinal cord running from the brain stem to the first or second lumbar vertebrae.

Cause of injury

Improper weight lifting technique. Excessive strain. Forceful trauma to the vertebral disc.

Signs and symptoms

Pain in the back or neck. Numbness, tingling, or pain in the buttocks, back, legs, or feet. Difficulty controlling bowel or bladder.

Complications if left unattended

Slipped or herniated discs require medical attention and evaluation. Symptoms of slipped disc may indicate other underlying ailments including fracture, tumours, infection or nerve damage, with serious—in certain cases, life-threatening—implications.

Immediate treatment

Bed rest, application of alternating ice and heat. Use of anti-inflammatory and pain relieving medications.

Rehabilitation and prevention

Bed rest and limited activity for several days is usually indicated, though normal, non-athletic daily activity should be resumed soon thereafter, to prevent atrophy and restore mobility in the spine. Physical therapy may be combined with massage and gradually increasing exercise of the back, after the pain has subsided. Strengthening and flexibility exercises, proper warm-up, avoidance of excessive or sudden weight lifting and attention to good sports technique may help avoid the injury.

Long-term prognosis

Most disc injuries are resolved without surgery, given proper recovery time. Though full restoration of strength and mobility may generally be expected, discs are vulnerable to re-injury, particularly for weight lifters and athletes placing significant demands on the back muscles, tendons, and ligaments and on the spine itself.

Brief outline of injury

Discs are segments of connective tissue that separate the vertebrae of the spine, providing absorption from shock and allowing for the smooth flexing of the neck and back without the vertebral bones rubbing against each other. A bulging disc is one that has extended outward beyond its normal boundary, due to various forms of degeneration. Should the disc impinge on the ligaments connecting the vertebrae or on nerves of the spine, pain results, though the affliction can also be painless in many cases.

Anatomy and physiology

The spine is made up of bones known as *vertebrae*, separated by fibrocartilaginous intervertebral discs. There is only slight movement between any two successive vertebrae, but there is considerable movement *through* the spinal column. The intervertebral discs are composed of a thick ring of fibrous cartilage, known as the *annulus fibrosis* which surrounds a jelly-like material known as the *nucleus pulposus*, and provide flexibility, cushioning, and protection to the spine. The *spinal canal* runs through the center of the vertebrae and discs and contains the spinal cord running from the brain stem to the first or second lumbar vertebrae. A bulging disc may result when the nucleus pulposus pushes outward.

Cause of injury

Age-related wear and degeneration. Stretching of ligaments connecting vertebrae. Successive strain from improper weight training.

Signs and symptoms

Back pain radiating to the legs (lumbar discs). Back pain radiating to the shoulders (cervical discs). Asymptomatic, only appearing on a magnetic resonance imaging (MRI) scan.

Complications if left unattended

A bulging disc may not cause pain or other symptoms and may not be recognized without a medical scan. As a disc bulges more over time however, it may begin to impinge on nerves and cause pain. Sudden stress to the discs, as during abrupt movements or weight lifting, can cause rupture or herniation of the discs, a more painful condition requiring rest and rehabilitation.

Immediate treatment

Cessation of activity stressing the spinal discs. Rest and alternating ice and heat to reduce inflammation and pain.

Rehabilitation and prevention

Bulging discs often occur as a natural consequence of the aging process, though in some cases, they are a precursor to herniation or rupture of the disc, with the leakage of the disc's gel-like center. Bulging discs are an example of *contained* injury while herniated discs are considered *uncontained*. Minimizing undue stress on the back may help avoid this injury.

Long-term prognosis

More severely bulging discs may in time rupture, causing the inner material to extrude into the spinal canal. In less severe cases, rest and ice are generally sufficient to restore pain-free mobility to the athlete.

Rehabilitation exercises

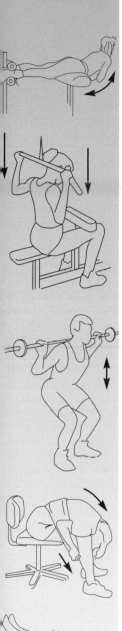

Brief outline of injury

Stress fractures of the vertebrae (*spondylolysis*) are a common athletic injury, caused by overuse or hyperextension of the spine. Gymnastics, weight lifting, and football are among the sports prone to this injury. Stress fractures most often occur in the fifth lumbar vertebra and act to weaken the bone, sometimes to the point where the vertebrae shift out of place; this condition is known as *spondylolisthesis*.

Anatomy and physiology

The upper and lower joints of the lumbar spine are joined by the *pars interarticularis*, the weakest bony portion of the vertebral neural arch, and the region between the superior and inferior articular facets. Overuse injuries can result in cracks or fractures in the pars interarticularis, a particularly common occurrence in adolescent athletes during sudden growth spurts. The lowest lumbar vertebra (L5), where the spine meets the pelvis, is the most common site for vertebral fractures.

Cause of injury

Genetic predisposition. Mechanical stress caused by overuse, flexion, twisting, or hyperextension of the lumbar spine. Growth spurts, especially in adolescents.

Signs and symptoms

Pain spreading across the lower back. Spasms causing stiffening in the back. Tightening of hamstring muscles, causing changes in posture.

Complications if left unattended

If slippage due to vertebral fracturing is ignored, it will worsen and can become incapacitating. Bone that has developed cracks requires sufficient time to rebuild, a process known as *remodeling*. Surgery may ultimately be required should fractures further develop and become severe.

Immediate treatment

Rest and avoidance of overuse or stress to the lumbar vertebrae. Ice pack, analgesic and anti-inflammatory drugs to reduce inflammation and pain. Then heat to promote blood flow and healing.

Rehabilitation and prevention

Following a thorough healing period (which may last 6 weeks or longer depending on the severity of injury), flexibility and strength training exercises should be undertaken, avoiding overuse. Exercising on hard, inflexible surfaces like concrete increases the forces causing stress to the lumbar spine, and should likewise be avoided.

Long-term prognosis

Unlike most stress fractures, spondylolysis (and spondylolisthesis) do not typically heal with time, although given adequate healing time, bone remodeling tends to repair lumbar fractures, particularly in less severe cases. Should rest and normal rehabilitation fail to restore mobility and should long-term pain persist, spinal surgery (in which the lumbar vertebrae are fused with the sacrum) may be necessary.

Chapter

11

Sports Injuries of the
Chest and
Abdomen

Acute

060: Broken (Fractured) Ribs

061: Flail Chest

062: Abdominal Muscle Strain

a)

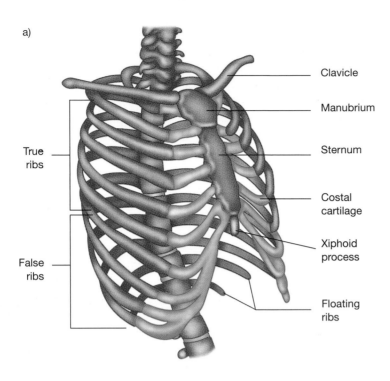

Clavicle

Manubrium

Sternum

Costal cartilage

Xiphoid process

Floating ribs

True ribs

False ribs

b)

Ribs elevate and sternum contracts

Lung

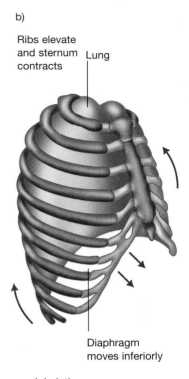

Diaphragm moves inferiorly

Inhalation

Figure 11.1: a) The ribs and sternum, b) the mechanics of respiration.

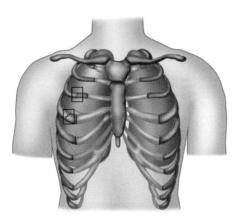

Broken or fractured ribs

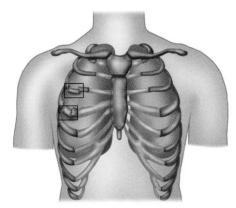

Flail chest

Lung

Ribs and sternum depress

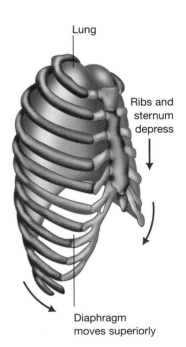

Diaphragm moves superiorly

Exhalation

**Rehabilitation
exercises**

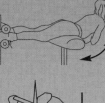

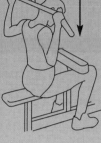

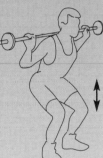

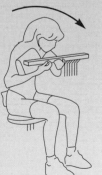

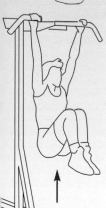

Brief outline of injury

Contact sports such as football and hockey, or sports that may result in falls or blunt trauma to the chest have a higher incidence of rib fractures than other sports. Extreme sports, horseback riding, and martial arts are other examples of activities that may result in this injury. Pain and tenderness over the rib cage after blunt trauma or a fall, especially with difficulty breathing, should always be treated as potentially broken ribs, and medical help sought.

Anatomy and physiology

There are twelve pairs of ribs, comprising true, false, and floating ribs. The first seven pairs are known as *true ribs*, and attach by costal cartilage directly to the sternum. The next *three* pairs are known as the false ribs, and attach to costal cartilage but not directly to the sternum. The final two pairs of ribs are known as *floating ribs*, and lack attachment either to costal cartilage or to the sternum.

The ribs protect the organs inside the chest (thoracic) cavity, and are also essential in the breathing mechanism. The muscles responsible for opening up the chest cavity, to allow air to enter the lungs, attach to the ribs. The ribs are more flexible than many other bones due to their cartilaginous attachments. When the ribs or the cartilage attachments fracture or break, they weaken the support and protection of the chest cavity. This also interferes with the muscles' ability to open the chest cavity effectively to allow for adequate ventilation, which results in poor air intake and oxygen exchange. Any of the ribs may fracture, and often more than one rib is involved in the injury.

Cause of injury

Hard blow to the chest, side, or back. Fall, landing on the chest, back or side. Forceful coughing – most common in people with impaired bone health, e.g. osteoporosis.

Signs and symptoms

Pain and tenderness over the fracture site, which may be noted also when pressing on the sternum or compressing the rib cage. Pain and difficulty breathing, especially on inhalation. Depending on the number of ribs involved, irregular movement of the chest during respirations may be noted, as well as some swelling.

Complications if left unattended

Fractured ribs that are left unattended will be painful and could lead to infections in the lungs due to shallow breathing. Reduced oxygen levels may result from the lower volume of air taken in. The bone ends may separate and cause damage to the delicate lung tissue underneath, causing a punctured lung or other damage; possibly even to the heart. Overall stability of the chest cavity will be affected also.

Immediate treatment

If a rib fracture is suspected, seek medical attention. Ice and anti-inflammatory medication may be used for pain relief. Compression may be used to stabilize the area until medical help is obtained, but should not be used long-term due to the limiting of deep, cleansing breaths needed for lung tissue health.

Rehabilitation and prevention

Rest is essential for recovery and repair of fractured ribs. It is important to take at least one deep, lung expanding breath each hour to ensure adequate lung tissue involvement and avoid infections in the lungs. Protecting the injured area until it is completely healed is important. Due to the inability to totally rest this area because of its constant movement during respirations, it takes longer to heal, usually 6–8 weeks. When returning to activity, this area should be padded and protected for an additional week or two.

Building muscle mass in the chest and back will help protect the ribs from injury. Using properly fitting and appropriate protective equipment will help to protect the ribs also. Avoiding trauma to the rib cage is the most important step in preventing rib fractures.

Long-term prognosis

Ribs usually heal completely if given adequate rest. The chances of breaking a rib are no greater after an initial break, if it is allowed to heal completely. The number of ribs involved in the injury may impact overall recovery time. If underlying tissue, such as the heart or lungs, is involved in the injury it may take much longer to heal completely and therefore may result in significant recovery time.

Rehabilitation exercises

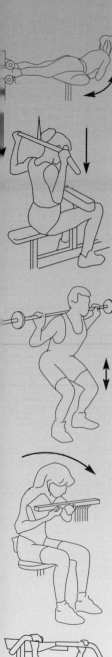

Brief outline of injury

When ribs are fractured in multiple places allowing portions to float free, flail chest may result. The chest wall is no longer one unit and the detached area may move separately from the rest of the chest wall. This is a serious condition due to the delicate nature of the underlying organs and the role of the ribs, and chest wall, in the process of breathing. This is a medical emergency and should be treated immediately.

Anatomy and physiology

The ribs form a cage that protects the thoracic cavity. When a rib is broken in two or more places, the integrity of the cage fails, and the chest wall loses its rigid support. This is especially true when more than one rib is involved in the injury. This may also occur when the cartilage is broken along with a fracture in the rib itself. The ability of the chest to expand and move air into, and out of, the lungs is affected and respirations become irregular and shallow. Paradoxical chest rise or uneven rise across the entire chest cavity, often accompanies this injury. It is usually seen as opposite from normal respiratory rise, resulting in the chest collapsing during inhalation and expanding during exhalation.

Cause of injury

Blunt trauma to the rib cage. Fall or other direct blow to the chest, back, or side. Crush injury to the thoracic area. Untreated rib fracture with additional trauma.

Signs and symptoms

Unequal or uneven chest rise. One area may seem to move independent of the rest of the chest and in opposition to normal respiratory rise. Pain and tenderness. Difficulty breathing. Bruising, and possible swelling, over the injured area. Instability in the chest wall over the fractured ribs.

Complications if left unattended

In flail chest, the broken ribs are floating free and therefore prone to cause injury to the delicate lung and heart tissue immediately below. This could lead to a *pneumothorax* (air in the chest cavity, outside the lungs) or *haemothorax* (loss of blood into the pleural cavity, but outside the lungs). Adequate breathing is affected by the pain and instability associated with this injury as well. The inability to produce quality respirations could lead to *hypoxia* (a reduced concentration of oxygen in air, blood, or tissue). The inability to fully inflate the lungs could lead to pneumonia and other respiratory complications.

Immediate treatment

This injury is a medical emergency due to the possible complications, and immediate medical help should be sought. Ice and anti-inflammatory or pain medication may be used for pain management. Compression of the injured area for stabilization may be used until medical help is obtained, but should not be used long-term due to the compromising of proper ventilation of the lungs.

Rehabilitation and prevention

Rest is the most important step in the recovery phase of this injury. Protecting the injured area is important as well. Return to activity should be slow and the injured area padded for additional protection. The muscles surrounding the injury site will require rehabilitation when the fractures have healed. This should be approached cautiously and gradually.

Strengthening and building muscle mass around the rib cage will help protect it from injury. The thick muscles of the chest and back provide good protection. The side of the rib cage should be protected with protective gear. Avoiding trauma to the rib cage will also reduce the chances of this injury.

Long-term prognosis

Flail chest should recover fully with adequate rest and rehabilitation. In some cases surgical intervention may be required to stabilize the fractured ribs. When many ribs are involved, or multiple fractures are found in each rib, the recovery time will be increased. Damage to the underlying tissue, or to supportive tissues, may increase the overall healing time as well.

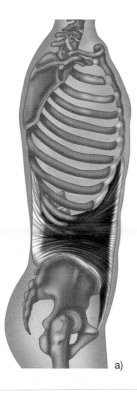 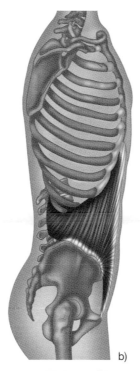 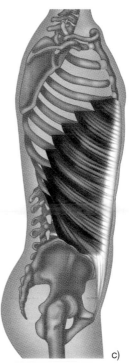

a) b) c)

Figure 11.2: Muscles of the abdomen; a) transversus abdominis, b) internal oblique, c) external oblique, d) rectus abdominis.

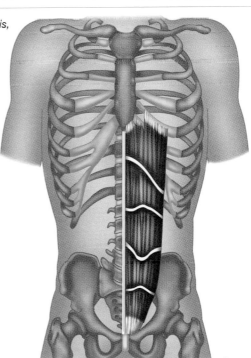

d)

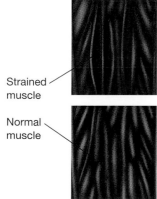

Strained muscle

Normal muscle

Muscle strain

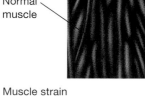

062: ABDOMINAL MUSCLE STRAIN

Brief outline of injury

Strains are injuries to a muscle or tendon. Strain to the abdominal muscle (also known as a *pulled abdominal muscle*) occurs from overstretching and/or tearing of muscle fibres, a common injury in many sports. Such tearing tends to be mild but in severe cases, the muscle can rupture.

Anatomy and physiology

The anterior abdominal wall muscles occur between the ribs and the pelvis, encircling the internal organs, and act to support the trunk, permit movement, hold the organs in place, and support the lower back. There are three layers of muscle, with fibres running in the same direction as the corresponding three layers of muscle in the thoracic wall. The deepest layer consists of the *transversus abdominis*, whose fibres run approximately horizontally. The middle layer comprises the *internal oblique*, whose fibres are crossed by the outermost layer known as the *external oblique*, forming a pattern of fibres resembling a St. Andrew's cross. Overlying these three layers is the *rectus abdominis*, which runs vertically, either side of the midline of the abdomen, and is associated with the *six-pack* muscles seen in conditioned athletes.

Cause of injury

Muscle stretched too far. Muscle stretched while contracting. Sudden, violent movement of the trunk. Direct trauma.

Signs and symptoms

Abdominal pain at the injured muscle. Lower back pain. Muscle spasms, occasionally bruising.

Complications if left unattended

Muscle strains of the abdomen are common and usually resolve themselves with rest, although continued vigorous exercise and inadequate healing time can lead to more serious tearing of muscle and tendon, damage to these structures, prolonged pain, and interference with normal activity.

Immediate treatment

R.I.C.E.R. regimen to reduce inflammation and treat pain. Anti-inflammatory medication and standard analgesics.

Rehabilitation and prevention

Rest and adequate healing time are generally sufficient to relieve muscle strains of the abdomen and return the athlete to full capacity. Targeted exercises to strengthen the abdominal muscles, including slow repetition exercises for abdomen and spine, may then be undertaken. Attention to proper technique is critical in avoiding muscle strain injuries, as is thorough stretching prior to sports activity.

Long-term prognosis

Abdominal muscle strains broadly fall into three categories of severity, each requiring similar care but varying lengths of time for proper healing. Generally, a full recovery to normal sports activity can be expected. The condition occurring without serious complication does not require surgery.

Rehabilitation exercises

Chapter

12

Sports Injuries of the
Hips, Pelvis,
and Groin

Acute

063: Hip Flexor Strain

064: Hip Pointer

065: Avulsion Fracture

066: Groin Strain

Chronic

067: Osteitis Pubis

068: Stress Fracture

069: Piriformis Syndrome

070: Iliopsoas Tendinitis

071: Tendinitis of the Adductor Muscles

072: Snapping Hip Syndrome

073: Trochanteric Bursitis

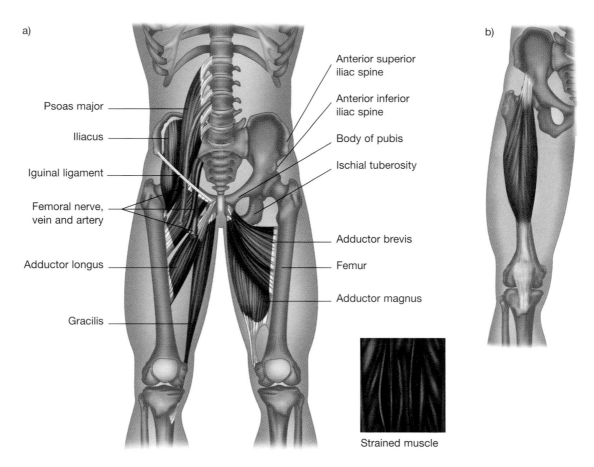

a)

Psoas major

Iliacus

Iguinal ligament

Femoral nerve,
vein and artery

Adductor longus

Gracilis

Anterior superior
iliac spine

Anterior inferior
iliac spine

Body of pubis

Ischial tuberosity

Adductor brevis

Femur

Adductor magnus

b)

Strained muscle

Figure 12.1: The iliopsoas, adductors, and pelvic region, anterior view, b) the rectus femoris muscle, posterior view.

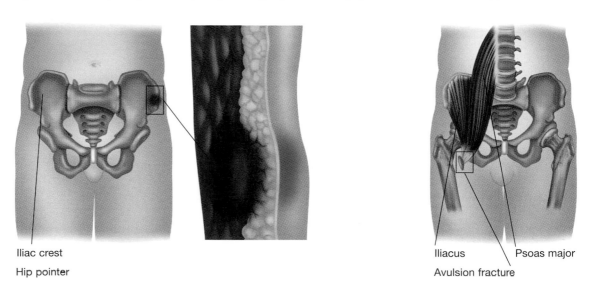

Iliac crest

Hip pointer

Iliacus

Psoas major

Avulsion fracture

**Rehabilitation
exercises**

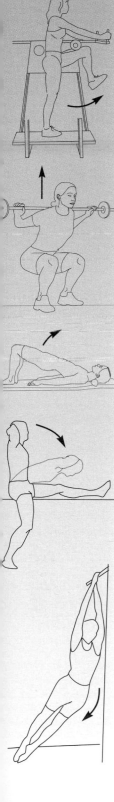

Brief outline of injury

A strain is a stretch or tear of a muscle or tendon. The hip flexor is a muscle located on the front of the hip that lifts the upper leg forward and upward or bends the waist forward when flexed. This muscle is used a lot in cycling, running, kicking, and jumping activities. When a new load is placed on the muscle or repetitive stresses are encountered without rest, the muscle may stretch or tear.

Anatomy and physiology

The hip flexor is made up of the *iliopsoas* (the iliacus and the psoas major) and the *rectus femoris*. These muscles attach to the hip on their upper attachment and the femur on the lower attachment. Their function is to pull the femur toward the abdomen, or conversely to pull the abdomen toward the legs, as in a sit-up. Runners, cyclists, soccer players, hikers, and people involved in jumping activities where the legs are lifted are all at risk of hip flexor strains.

Cause of injury

Repetitive stress on the hip flexor muscles without adequate rest for recovery. Excessive stress placed on the muscle without appropriate strengthening and warm-up. Improper form when running, cycling or other activities that involve the hip flexors. Forceful hyperextension of the leg at the hip.

Signs and symptoms

Pain in the upper groin area over the anterior portion of the hip. Pain with movement of the leg at the hip. Inflammation and tenderness over the hip flexor.

Complications if left unattended

Hip flexor strains left untreated can become chronic and lead to inflexible muscles that could lead to other disorders. The muscle could also continue to tear, eventually leading to a complete tearing away from the attachment.

Immediate treatment

Cessation of activities that aggravate the hip flexors. Ice for the first 48–72 hours. Anti-inflammatory drugs. Then heat and massage to promote blood flow and healing.

Rehabilitation and prevention

Conditioning is the key to rehabilitation and prevention of hip flexor strains. Muscles that are strong and flexible are much more resilient. Stretching the hip flexors, abdominals, lower back, quadriceps, and hamstrings helps to lower the stress load placed on the hip flexors. Strengthening of the iliopsoas and the other muscles of the hip, quadriceps, lower back, and abdomen will help to prepare the hip flexors for unexpected stresses.

Long-term prognosis

Although the potential for chronic pain and inflexibility exists, hip flexor strains usually recover fully when given adequate rest and then active recovery using stretching and strengthening.

Brief outline of injury

The hip pointer usually refers to a deep bruise of the iliac crest and the muscles that cover it, and is often caused by a direct blow. Hip pointers are most commonly associated with football but may be seen in any contact sport.

Anatomy and physiology

A hip pointer is usually a bruise of the muscle or bone, but can be as severe as a chip or fracture. The iliac crest (commonly referred to as the *hip bone*), felt when you rest your hands on your hips, is the bone involved, and the muscles that attach to the iliac crest include the hip flexors, the abdominals, and the muscles responsible for the rotation of the hips. Because these muscles are injured at their attachments, any movement involving these muscles will be painful.

Cause of injury

Direct impact to the hip.

Signs and symptoms

Pain and tenderness over the iliac crest. Pain with movement of the hip, and sometimes with weight bearing (due to the muscle involvement). Inflammation in the hip area.

Complications if left unattended

Left unattended, the pain and inflammation can lead to improper gait and become chronic. If the bone is chipped or fractured, failure to treat can lead to improper healing and future injuries to the site.

Immediate treatment

Removal from the activity. Ice the area immediately. X-ray for possible fracture.

Rehabilitation and prevention

Preventing hip pointers includes proper protective equipment during activities, and strengthening the supporting muscles around the hip for added padding and protection. Unfortunately there is not a lot that can be done to prevent falling or contact to the hip area.

Rehabilitation includes rest until the pain subsides, then gradual reintroduction into the activity. Any activities causing pain should be discontinued until it is pain free.

Long-term prognosis

Hip pointers seldom cause long-term disability and most athletes can return to full function after treatment and a rehabilitation period. Surgery is seldom required except in severe fracture cases.

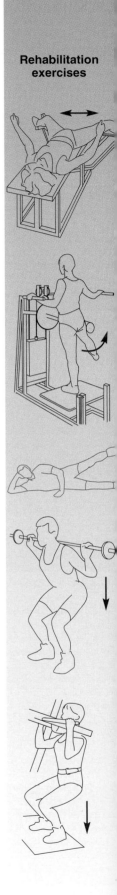

Rehabilitation exercises

065: AVULSION FRACTURE

Rehabilitation exercises

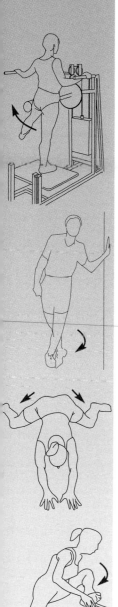

Brief outline of injury

An avulsion fracture occurs when a tendon or ligament pulls away from the bone at its attachment, pulling a piece of the bone away with it. This usually results from a forceful twisting muscular contraction, or powerful hyperextension or hyperflexion. This injury is more prevalent in children than in adults. The tendon or ligament tends to tear before the bone is involved in adults, but the softer bones tend to become involved in children. Most commonly seen in boys between 13 and 17, although the ligament-bone junction is a common site of injury in middle-aged people.

Anatomy and physiology

Although any tendon or ligament in the body can be involved in an avulsion fracture, it is more common in those around the *pelvis*. Avulsion fractures most commonly occur at *apophyses*, sites where a major tendon attaches onto a growing bony prominence. In children, the *growth plate* is a weaker site where the bone is continuously forming, and is an area where avulsion fractures often occur. The anterior superior iliac spine, the anterior inferior iliac spine, and the ischial tuberosity are the bony prominences most commonly involved. The corresponding muscles affected are the sartorius, the rectus femoris and the hamstrings (see page 176), respectively. If a musculo-tendinous unit is involved, muscle function will be limited.

Cause of injury

Forceful twisting, extending, or flexing causing extra stress on the ligaments or tendons. Direct impact on a joint causing forceful stretching of the ligaments.

Signs and symptoms

Pain, swelling, and tenderness at the injury site. Sudden localized pain that may radiate down the muscle.

Complications if left unattended

When left untreated, an avulsion fracture will lead to long-term disability in the muscles and joints involved. Incomplete, or incorrect healing may result as well, leading to future injuries to other muscles.

Immediate treatment

R.I.C.E.R. treatment. Immobilization of the joint involved. Anti-inflammatory drugs. Seek immediate medical help.

Rehabilitation and prevention

Rest for the injured muscles and joints, and then strengthening of the muscles and supporting ligaments, will help rehabilitate and prevent future fractures. Gradual re-entry into full activity is important to prevent re-injuring the weakened area.

Long-term prognosis

With proper treatment, most simple avulsion fractures will heal completely with no limitations. In rare cases surgery may be needed to repair the avulsed bone, especially in children when the avulsion involves a growth plate.

SPORTS INJURIES OF THE HIPS, PELVIS, AND GROIN

066: GROIN STRAIN

Brief outline of injury

As with any strain, the groin strain (also known as *rider's strain*) is a stretch or tear of any or all of the adductor muscles of the inner thigh or their tendons. Soccer, hockey and other sports that require pivoting and quick direction changes are the most common activities for groin pulls. These injuries range from simple stretching of the muscles to more severe tearing of the fibres. As with other strains it is graded 1 through to 3 with 3 being the most severe tear.

Anatomy and physiology

The groin area covers the inner thigh. The muscles involved include the pectineus, adductor brevis, adductor longus, gracilis and adductor magnus. These muscles are responsible for pulling the leg in toward the midline of the body, and attach at the pelvis and the femur, some up high and others closer to the knee. Due to this location and function, athletes involved in sports where the leg is moved forcefully inward or outward are more susceptible to this injury. Damage is usually to the musculo-tendinous junction, about 5 cm from the pubis.

Cause of injury

Forceful stretching of the adductor muscles of the hip. Forceful contraction of the adductor muscles.

Signs and symptoms

Grade 1: Mild pain, stiffness in the adductor muscles, and little or no effect on athletic performance.
Grade 2: More painful, swelling, tenderness, limited range of motion, pain when walking or jogging.
Grade 3: Very painful, a lot of swelling, pain with weight bearing, sometimes pain at rest or at night.

Complications if left unattended

Untreated groin strains can lead to an awkward gait and chronic pain that could lead to injuries in other areas. A minor muscle tear could become more severe and eventually tear completely.

Immediate treatment

R.I.C.E.R. immediately. Anti-inflammatory medication. For a *Grade 3 strain* it may be necessary to seek a medical evaluation.

Rehabilitation and prevention

After initial treatment, minor strains will respond to a gradual stretching and strengthening program. More serious strains will require additional rest and a slow entry back into activities with extra warm-up activities before each session.

Prevention of groin strains requires warming-up properly before activities, stretching for good flexibility in the adductors and strengthening of the abductor muscles, adductor muscles, abdominals, and hip flexors for good muscular balance.

Long-term prognosis

Most groin strains will heal with no lingering effects. Only the most severe strains, with complete tears, require surgical correction.

Rehabilitation exercises

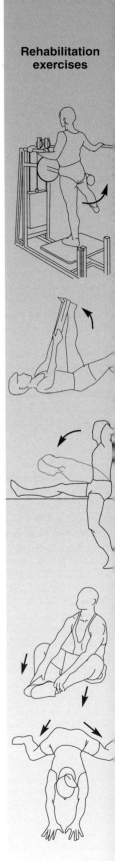

a)

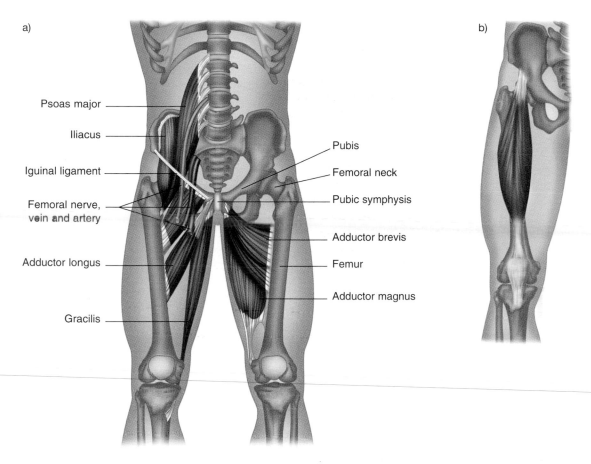

Psoas major

Iliacus

Iguinal ligament

Femoral nerve, vein and artery

Adductor longus

Gracilis

Pubis

Femoral neck

Pubic symphysis

Adductor brevis

Femur

Adductor magnus

b)

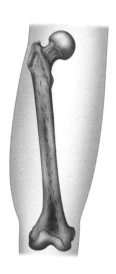

Figure 12.2: The iliopsoas, adductors, and pelvic region, anterior view, b) the rectus femoris muscle, posterior view.

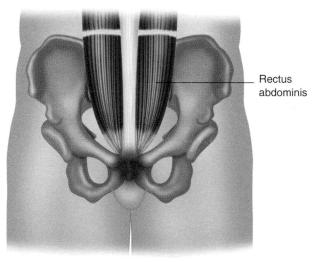

Rectus abdominis

Osteitis pubis

Stress fracture

Brief outline of injury

Osteitis pubis is an inflammation of the pubic symphysis and the surrounding muscles. This is a chronic problem that often results from a muscle imbalance, repetitive stresses, or an untreated injury to the bones or musculature of the area. Soccer players, hockey players, sprinters and other athletes who are involved in running, kicking or rapid lateral movement are more susceptible to this type of injury.

Anatomy and physiology

The pelvis, more specifically the *pubic symphysis*, a fibrocartilage disc, is involved in this injury. No instability of the pubic symphysis occurs, but there is tenderness over the area. The adductor muscles of the hips and the hip flexors are also involved. Repetitive stresses on this area or a change in the angle of stress, from a major trauma, can lead to a change in the structure of the pubic symphysis. This causes a shift in the pull of the muscles attached there.

Cause of injury

Repetitive stresses on the pubic symphysis from running, kicking, etc. Unresolved trauma to this area resulting in abnormal forces on the pubic symphysis.

Signs and symptoms

Adductor or lower abdomen pain that localizes to the pubic area. Pain increases with running, kicking, or pushing off to change direction.

Complications if left unattended

Untreated osteitis pubis will lead to increased pain and disability. The increased pain may lead to awkward form during certain activities that could lead to other injuries.

Immediate treatment

Ice and rest from offending activities. Anti-inflammatory medication.

Rehabilitation and prevention

Restoring flexibility to the entire hip girdle is important when the pain subsides. Gradual involvement in the athletic activities is also important. Stop an activity if it causes pain. Strengthening the adductor muscles and the hip flexors also prepares this area to handle the stresses more efficiently. Proper warm-up techniques before running, kicking or other direct impact activities are important as well.

Long-term prognosis

When treated properly, there are seldom any long-term effects. Full range of motion and strength should return. If pain and limited mobility linger, the injury should be re-evaluated.

Rehabilitation exercises

Brief outline of injury

Repetitive stress or unnatural stress placed on the surface of a bone, often from muscle fatigue, can lead to stress fractures. Running, jumping, and other high impact activities can lead to small cracks or fractures along a bone. Stress fractures can occur in any bone subjected to repetitive stress or impact.

Anatomy and physiology

Stress fractures can occur in any bone but are most commonly found in the bones of the foot, lower leg, and hip. When a muscle becomes fatigued and can no longer absorb the shock of impact, that stress gets transferred to the bone. Over time that stress will cause small cracks in the bone. Fatigue in certain muscles may also create strength imbalances that put an unnatural stress on the bone causing small fractures. Stress fractures to the pubis, femoral neck, and proximal third of the femur are seen in individuals who perform aerobic dance activities, or extensive jogging.

Cause of injury

Repetitive stress from impact activities. Unnatural stress on a bone from different running surfaces. Strength imbalances causing unusual stress.

Signs and symptoms

Generalized area of pain. Pain with weight bearing. When running, the pain is severe in the beginning, then none-to-moderate pain in the middle, with severe pain returning at the end and after the run.

Complications if left unattended

When left unattended a stress fracture may develop into a more serious complete fracture. The pain and natural guarding of the injured area could lead to future injuries in other areas.

Immediate treatment

Rest is the most important treatment. Anti-inflammatory drugs.

Rehabilitation and prevention

When rehabbing a stress fracture it is important to start activity slowly. It may take 4–8 weeks for a fracture to completely heal. During that time it is important to identify training problems that may have caused the stress fracture originally. It is also important during this time to keep up general conditioning using activities that do not require excessive impact on the affected area.

To prevent stress fractures, it is important to warm-up properly before activities, and use proper equipment (avoid using worn out running shoes, etc.). It is also important to increase intensity slowly and eat plenty of calcium-rich foods.

Long-term prognosis

With proper treatment and rehabilitation most stress fractures heal completely with no future concerns. A very rare few may require surgical pinning to strengthen the fracture area.

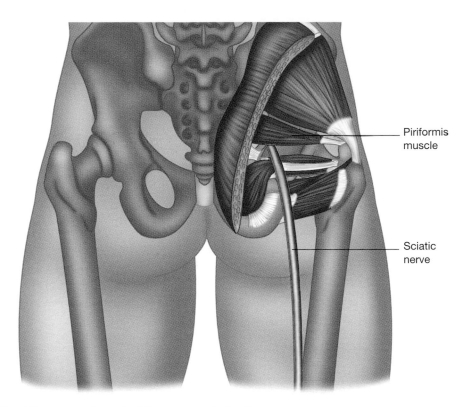

Piriformis
muscle

Sciatic
nerve

Figure 12.3a: The piriformis muscle, and sciatic nerve, posterior view.

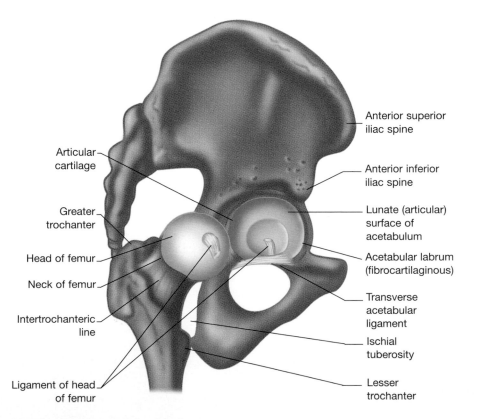

Anterior superior
iliac spine

Anterior inferior
iliac spine

Lunate (articular)
surface of
acetabulum

Acetabular labrum
(fibrocartilaginous)

Transverse
acetabular
ligament

Ischial
tuberosity

Lesser
trochanter

Articular
cartilage

Greater
trochanter

Head of femur

Neck of femur

Intertrochanteric
line

Ligament of head
of femur

Figure 12.3b: The hip joint, right leg, lateral view.

069: PIRIFORMIS SYNDROME

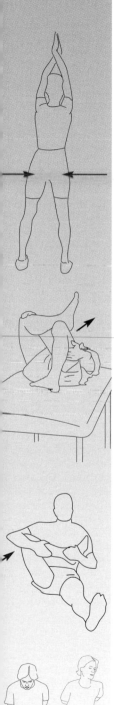

Brief outline of injury

Piriformis syndrome is a result of pressure applied to the sciatic nerve by the piriformis muscle. The pain usually runs from the buttocks down to the back of the thigh. Incorrect form or improper gait often leads to tightness and inflexibility in this muscle. This condition occurs more frequently in women than men (6:1).

Anatomy and physiology

The piriformis muscle is a small, tubular muscle that originates at the internal surface of the sacrum, inserts at the superior border of the greater trochanter of the femur, and leaves the pelvis by passing through the greater sciatic foramen. The muscle assists in laterally rotating the hip joint, abducting the thigh when the hip is flexed, and helps to hold the head of the femur in the *acetabulum*. When the muscle becomes tight, it puts pressure on the underlying nerve, causing pain similar to sciatica. The pain usually starts in the mid-buttocks region and radiates down through the hamstrings.

Cause of injury

Incorrect form or gait while walking or jogging. Weak abductor muscles and/or tight adductor muscles.

Signs and symptoms

Pain along the sciatic nerve. Pain when climbing stairs or walking up an incline. Increased pain after prolonged sitting.

Complications if left unattended

Chronic pain will result if left untreated. The tight muscle could also become irritated causing stress on the tendons and attachments.

Immediate treatment

R.I.C.E.R. Anti-inflammatory medication. Then heat and massage to promote blood flow and healing.

Rehabilitation and prevention

During rehabilitation, a gradual return to activity and continued stretching of the hip muscles is essential. Starting with lower intensity or duration when returning to activities is wise. Identifying the factors that initiated the problem is also important. Strengthening the abductor muscles and increasing the flexibility of the adductors will help to alleviate some of the stress and prevent the piriformis from becoming tight. Maintaining a good stretching regimen to keep the piriformis muscle flexible will help, while dealing with the other issues.

Long-term prognosis

Piriformis syndrome seldom results in long-term problems when treated properly. Rarely, a corticosteroid injection or other invasive method may be required to alleviate the pain and tightness.

a)

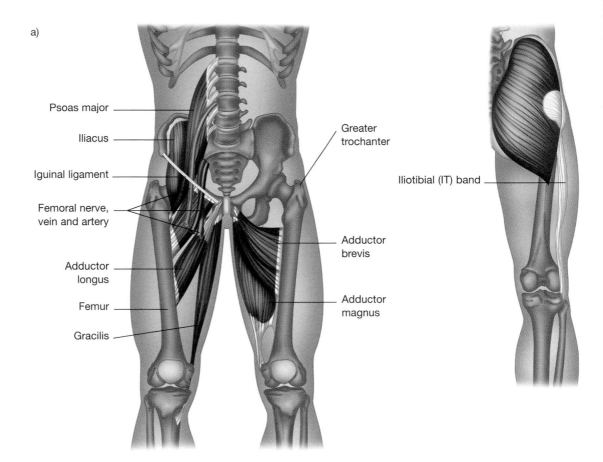

Psoas major

Iliacus

Iguinal ligament

Femoral nerve,
vein and artery

Adductor
longus

Femur

Gracilis

Greater
trochanter

Adductor
brevis

Adductor
magnus

Figure 12.4: The iliopsoas and adductor muscles.

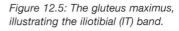

Iliotibial (IT) band

*Figure 12.5: The gluteus maximus,
illustrating the iliotibial (IT) band.*

Bone

Inflamed
tendon

Muscle

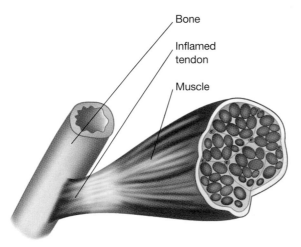

Tendinitis

070: ILIOPSOAS TENDINITIS

Rehabilitation exercises

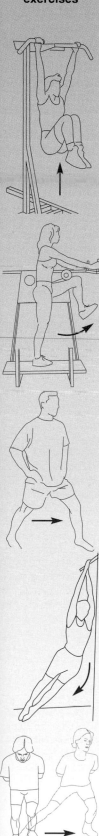

Brief outline of injury

Tendinitis is an inflammation of the tendon and connected muscle. It is usually caused by overuse or use of incorrect equipment. The iliopsoas muscle and tendon can become inflamed through repetitive hip flexion, such as is seen in running, jumping, and even weight training that involves a lot of bending and squatting.

Anatomy and physiology

The *iliopsoas* is actually made of two muscles; the iliacus, which originates at the hip bone, and the psoas major, which originates at the lumbar spine. Both muscles share their insertion at the top of the femur. The iliopsoas muscle is the main flexor of the hip joint. Repetitive flexion can cause inflammation of the tendon and muscle, and occasionally the underlying bursa.

Cause of injury

Repetitive hip flexion, such as running, jumping, and kicking. Untreated trauma to the iliopsoas muscle.

Signs and symptoms

Pain with hip movement. Tenderness over the upper groin area. Pain is gradual and worsens with activity.

Complications if left unattended

Tendinitis can eventually lead to a muscle tear if left untreated and the activity that caused it continues. Bursitis is also another problem that may develop from unattended tendinitis.

Immediate treatment

R.I.C.E.R. Anti-inflammatory medication. Then heat and massage to promote blood flow and healing.

Rehabilitation and prevention

Once most of the pain has been managed, it is important to start working on the strength and flexibility in the affected muscle. Increasing the flexibility in the opposing muscles responsible for hip extension, will help speed recovery and reduce the chance of recurrence. Proper warm-up before activity and developing a strength balance between hip flexors and extensors will also help prevent this injury.

Long-term prognosis

Iliopsoas tendinitis seldom needs more than the initial treatment and rehabilitation to recover fully. If pain persists or becomes more severe and sharp it may be necessary to consult a physician.

SPORTS INJURIES OF THE HIPS, PELVIS, AND GROIN

071: TENDINITIS OF THE ADDUCTOR MUSCLES

Brief outline of injury

Tendinitis is inflammation of a tendon or the tendon sheath. Inflammation to any, or all, of the five adductor muscles due to overuse can lead to pain in the groin area. Sprinting, playing football, hurdling and horseback riding can all cause overuse in these muscles. Unresolved injuries, such as a groin pull, can also lead to inflammation and pain in these muscles.

Anatomy and physiology

The adductor muscles, include the pectineus, adductor longus, adductor brevis, gracilis, and adductor magnus, and any of these may become inflamed. The pain is similar to a groin strain but is gradual and chronic in nature. The repetitive strain placed on these muscles from activities like sprinting can cause inflammation to the tendon and attached muscle.

Cause of injury

Repetitive stress to the adductor muscles. Previous injury, such as a groin strain. Tight abductor muscles.

Signs and symptoms

Pain in the groin area. Pain when pulling the legs together against resistance. Pain when running, especially sprinting.

Complications if left unattended

If left unattended, tendinitis to the adductor muscles can lead to injuries to the other muscles of the hip joint. It can also result in a tear of one or more of the adductor muscles.

Immediate treatment

Ice and rest from activities that cause pain. Anti-inflammatory medication. Then heat and massage to promote blood flow and healing.

Rehabilitation and prevention

Rehabilitation for tendinitis of the adductors starts with gradual reintroduction into activity with stretching and strengthening exercises for the affected muscles. It may be necessary to use heat packs on the affected area before exercise at first, and then continue with good warm-up activities to make sure the muscles are ready for the activity. Strengthening the adductors and stretching the opposing abductors will help prevent this injury from recurring. Treating all groin pulls and other hip injuries completely will also prevent problems with the adductors.

Long-term prognosis

Long-term problems are seldom seen with tendinitis of the adductor muscles after treatment. If pain and limited mobility in the hip persists, additional help may be required from a sports medicine specialist.

Rehabilitation exercises

072: SNAPPING HIP SYNDROME

Rehabilitation exercises

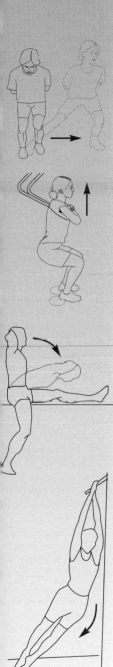

Brief outline of injury

Snapping hip syndrome is a condition where a *snapping* or *popping* sensation is felt in the hip with hip flexion and extension. There are a few possible causes for this, most commonly a tendon snapping over a bony prominence. Rarely, it can be from a tear in the cartilage of the hip joint. This syndrome may present with pain or not, and is particularly prevalent in dancers.

Anatomy and physiology

External snapping hip syndrome can be the result of a tight iliotibial (IT) band or gluteus maximus muscle snapping over the greater trochanter of the femur. When landing from a jump, running, climbing, or squatting these tendons are forced over the bony prominence of the greater trochanter. This causes inflammation of the muscle and tendon.

Internal snapping syndrome may be caused by the iliopsoas tendon snapping over the iliopectineal eminence of the hip. In more rare cases, tearing of the cartilage (labral tears) or loose bodies in the hip joint may cause snapping as well.

Cause of injury

Tight iliotibial band or buttock muscles. Tight iliopsoas muscle. Labral tear.

Signs and symptoms

Snapping sensation in the hip. May or may not present with pain (more commonly reported as discomfort).

Complications if left unattended

Snapping hip syndrome can lead to irritation, and possible rupture of the underlying bursa if left untreated. The inflamed muscle becomes tight and can cause stress on other muscles as well.

Immediate treatment

R.I.C.E.R. regimen. Anti-inflammatory medication.

Rehabilitation and prevention

Rehabilitation of snapping hip syndrome starts with stretching and strengthening the muscles of the hip. A balance in strength and flexibility of all the muscles will help prevent snapping hip syndrome. Proper warm-up of the hip muscles is important before beginning any activity that involves flexion or extension to make sure the muscles are adequately prepared for the activity. It is also important to maintain fitness levels while resting, using activities that do not aggravate the affected area.

Long-term prognosis

Snapping hip syndrome seldom requires more than the initial treatment and rehabilitation to recover fully. In very rare cases, surgical interventions may be required to correct the problem.

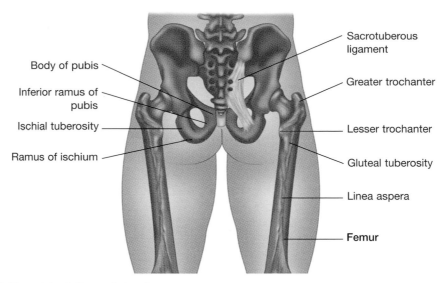

Body of pubis

Inferior ramus of pubis

Ischial tuberosity

Ramus of ischium

Sacrotuberous ligament

Greater trochanter

Lesser trochanter

Gluteal tuberosity

Linea aspera

Femur

Figure 12.6: The pelvic girdle, posterior view.

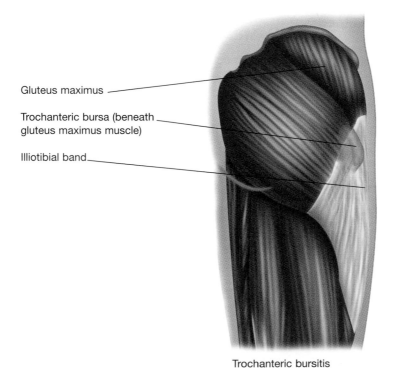

Gluteus maximus

Trochanteric bursa (beneath gluteus maximus muscle)

Illiotibial band

Trochanteric bursitis

Figure 12.7: The trochanteric bursa in relation to the greater trochanter, iliotibial (IT) band, and gluteus maximus.

Rehabilitation exercises

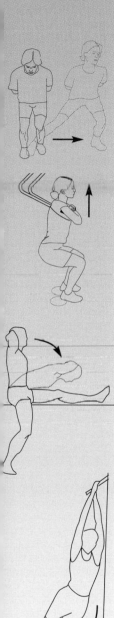

Brief outline of injury

A bursa is a fluid-filled sac that acts as a cushion to allow smooth movement between two rough surfaces. This commonly occurs between a bony prominence and a tendon or near the attachment of tendons. Trochanteric bursitis results when the bursa over the greater trochanter of the femur is irritated by repetitive stresses encountered during running activities.

Anatomy and physiology

The greater trochanter is the bony prominence on the upper portion of the femur to which some of the muscles of the hip and thigh attach. The *trochanteric bursa* lies between the gluteus maximus and the posterolateral surface of the greater trochanter. There are several muscles that cross this region, and because they are generally rubbing across the bone, the bursa can easily become inflamed. Because the greater trochanter is near the surface it is also susceptible to impact injuries. Also caused if the iliotibial band movement is limited.

Cause of injury

Repetitive hip activities such as running. Impact or other trauma to the bursa over the greater trochanter. Limited iliotibial band movement.

Signs and symptoms

Tenderness over the bony prominence of the upper thigh/hip. Swelling over the bursa. Pain when flexing or extending the hip, such as walking.

Complications if left unattended

If left unattended, this injury can cause chronic pain in the hip. The bursa may actually rupture with continued irritation to an already inflamed area.

Immediate treatment

Rest from offending activities. Ice. Anti-inflammatory medication.

Rehabilitation and prevention

Rest from the activities that aggravate the bursa is the first step in reducing pain and inflammation. After rest a gradual reintroduction is advised. Stop any activities that cause a recurrence of the pain. Creating a balance of strength and flexibility in all the muscles of the hip will help prevent trochanteric bursitis. Warming up the muscles of the hip properly before activity is also an important step in preventing this injury.

Long-term prognosis

Bursitis generally does not cause any long-term disability when treatment and rehabilitation programs are followed. Surgery is only a concern in very extreme cases.

Chapter

13

Sports Injuries of the
Hamstrings and
Quadriceps

Acute

074: Femur Fracture

075: Quadriceps Strain

076: Hamstring Strain

077: Thigh Bruise (Contusion)

Chronic

078: Iliotibial Band Syndrome

079: Quadriceps Tendinitis

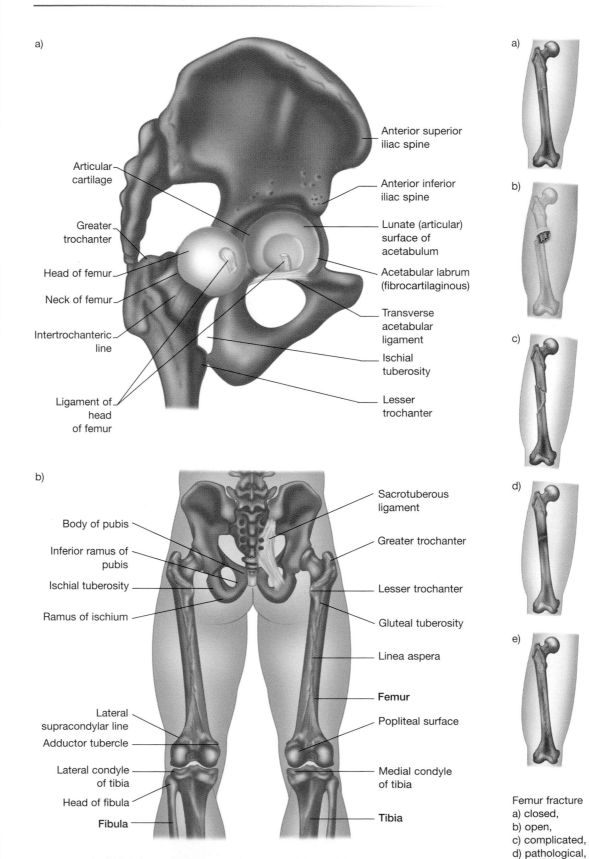

a)

Articular cartilage

Greater trochanter

Head of femur

Neck of femur

Intertrochanteric line

Ligament of head of femur

Anterior superior iliac spine

Anterior inferior iliac spine

Lunate (articular) surface of acetabulum

Acetabular labrum (fibrocartilaginous)

Transverse acetabular ligament

Ischial tuberosity

Lesser trochanter

b)

Body of pubis

Inferior ramus of pubis

Ischial tuberosity

Ramus of ischium

Lateral supracondylar line

Adductor tubercle

Lateral condyle of tibia

Head of fibula

Fibula

Sacrotuberous ligament

Greater trochanter

Lesser trochanter

Gluteal tuberosity

Linea aspera

Femur

Popliteal surface

Medial condyle of tibia

Tibia

a)

b)

c)

d)

e)

Femur fracture
a) closed,
b) open,
c) complicated,
d) pathological,
e) stress

Figure 13.1: The hip joint, a) right leg, lateral view, b) pelvic girdle to leg, posterior view.

Rehabilitation exercises

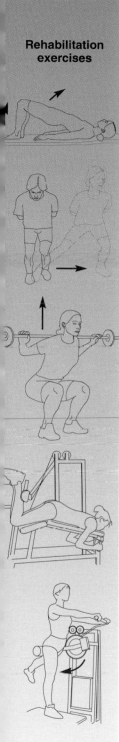

Brief outline of injury

It takes tremendous force to fracture the femur due to its strength, as well as the supporting musculature. Football, hockey, and other high impact sports are often associated with femur fractures.

Anatomy and physiology

The femur, also known as the *thigh bone*, is the heaviest, longest, and strongest bone in the body. Its proximal end has a ball-like head that articulates with the pelvic bone at the *acetabulum* and forms the hip joint. Distally are the *lateral* and *medial condyles*, which articulate with the tibia to form the *knee joint*. The quadriceps, hamstrings, adductor and abductor muscles surround the femur. The femur is more likely to fracture at the femoral neck, as it is smaller in diameter than the rest of the bone, and is composed of cancellous bone, which has a relatively low density. This would usually involve a hard impact, or excessive landing force from a high fall. The femur may also fracture along the shaft, which is usually caused by tremendous impact from a motor vehicle accident or sheering force across the femur.

Cause of injury

Super high impact across the femur, such as a car accident or aggressive tackle in football. High impact directed through the femur such as from landing from a high fall. Direct impact on the upper portion of the hip.

Signs and symptoms

Severe pain. Deformity and possible shortening of leg length. Swelling and discolouration. Inability to move the leg or bear weight.

Complications if left unattended

Permanent disability will result if this injury is left untreated. The large amount of blood loss due to internal injuries to the muscles and arteries could lead to shock and death.

Immediate treatment

Ice and immobilization. Seek immediate medical help.

Rehabilitation and prevention

Femur fractures involve extensive rehabilitation due to the time involved in healing and the musculature involved. The bone will most likely need to be surgically repaired with a plate, rod or pins, which increases the rehabilitation time. Rehabilitation will usually involve a physical therapist working on range of motion and strengthening of the muscles.

Prevention of a femur fracture requires avoiding activities that might result in high impact on the femur. Strengthening the muscles of the quadriceps, hamstrings, adductors, and abductors will also provide extra protection for the femur.

Long-term prognosis

With immediate treatment and repair of the femur along with rehabilitation to strengthen the supporting muscles, there should be no long-term limitations. Full recovery may take up to nine months.

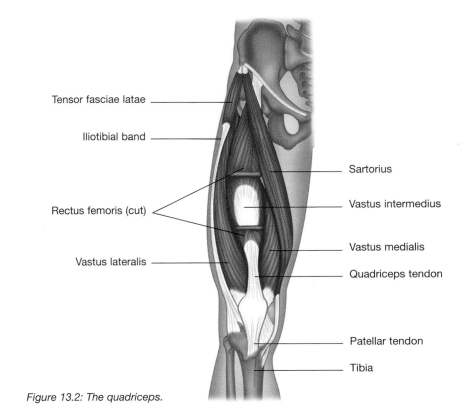

Tensor fasciae latae

Iliotibial band

Rectus femoris (cut)

Vastus lateralis

Sartorius

Vastus intermedius

Vastus medialis

Quadriceps tendon

Patellar tendon

Tibia

Figure 13.2: The quadriceps.

Strained muscle

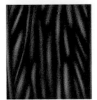

Normal muscle

Quadriceps and
Hamstring strain

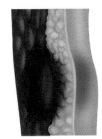

Thigh bruise
(contusion)

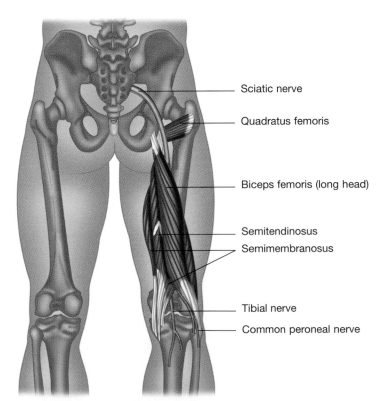

Sciatic nerve

Quadratus femoris

Biceps femoris (long head)

Semitendinosus
Semimembranosus

Tibial nerve

Common peroneal nerve

Figure 13.3: The hamstrings.

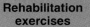

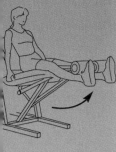

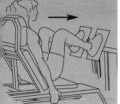

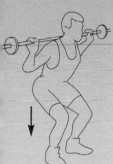

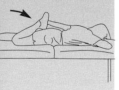

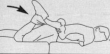

Brief outline of injury

A muscle strain, which is a forceful stretch or tear of the muscle or tendon in a weight bearing muscle such as the quadriceps, is painful and difficult to rest. The quadriceps are involved in supporting the hip and knee structure to hold the body weight. A quadriceps strain can result from a forceful contraction of the quadriceps or unusual stress placed on the muscles. As with other strains it is graded 1 through 3, with 3 being the most severe tear.

Anatomy and physiology

The *quadriceps* are composed of four muscles; the *vastus lateralis, vastus medialis, vastus intermedius,* and *rectus femoris*. A strain may occur in any of these muscles, but the *rectus femoris* is most commonly strained. Due to the force generated in activities such as sprinting, jumping, and weight training, the muscle may microtear, but when the muscle is stretched forcefully under a load such as with high impact sports like football and hockey, it may also pull away from the attachment or completely tear.

Cause of injury

Forceful contraction or stretch of the quadriceps.

Signs and symptoms

Grade 1: Mildly tender and painful, little or no swelling, full muscular strength.
Grade 2: More marked pain and tenderness, moderate swelling and possible bruising, noticeable strength loss.
Grade 3 (full tear): Extreme pain, deformity of the muscle, swelling and discolouration, inability to contract the muscle.

Complications if left unattended

A *grade 1 or 2* tear left unattended can continue to tear and become worse. A *grade 3* tear left untreated can result in loss of mobility and a severe loss of flexibility in the muscle.

Immediate treatment

R.I.C.E.R. Anti-inflammatory medication. Immobilization in severe cases. Then heat and massage to promote blood flow and healing.

Rehabilitation and prevention

After the required rest period, activities should be approached cautiously. Avoid activities that cause pain. Stretching and strengthening of the quadriceps will be necessary. Ensuring a balance of strength between the quadriceps and hamstrings is important to prevent a strain. Proper warm-up techniques must be observed to prevent strains and gradually increasing intensity will help as well.

Long-term prognosis

Quadriceps strains seldom result in long-term pain or disability. Surgery is only needed in rare cases where a complete tear does not respond to immobilization and rest.

Brief outline of injury

A hamstring strain, or a pulled hamstring as it is commonly referred to, is a stretch or tear of the hamstring muscles or tendons. This is a very common injury, especially in activities that involve sprinting or explosive accelerations. A common cause of a hamstring strain is a muscle imbalance between the hamstring and quadriceps, with the quadriceps being much stronger.

Anatomy and physiology

The hamstrings are three separate muscles that work together to extend the hip and flex the knee, and correspond to the flexors of the elbow in the upper limb. During running, the hamstrings slow down the leg at the end of its forward swing and prevent the trunk from flexing at the hip joint. The three muscles are the *biceps femoris, semitendinosus,* and the *semimembranosus*. Any of the muscles can be strained. Commonly minor tears happen in the belly of the muscle closest to the knee. Complete tears or ruptures usually pull away from this attachment as well. Excessive force against the muscles, especially during eccentric contraction (when the muscle is stretching against force), can cause stretching, minor tears, or even a complete rupture.

Cause of injury

Strength imbalance between the hamstrings and quadriceps. Forceful stretching of the muscle, especially during contraction. Excessive overload on the muscle.

Signs and symptoms

Pain and tenderness in the hamstrings; very little in a *grade 1*, to debilitating in a *grade 3*. May affect the ability to walk, from causing a limp, to a complete inability to bear weight. Swelling with *grades 2 and 3*.

Complications if left unattended

Pain and tightness in the hamstring will continue to get worse without treatment. The tightness in the hamstring could lead to lower back and hip problems. Untreated strains can continue to progress to a full rupture.

Immediate treatment

Grade 1: Ice, anti-inflammatory medicines.
Grades 2 and 3: R.I.C.E.R., anti-inflammatory medicines; seek medical help if a complete rupture is suspected or if the patient is unable to walk without aid. Then heat and massage to promote blood flow and healing.

Rehabilitation and prevention

Stretching after the initial pain subsides will help speed recovery and prevent future recurrences. Strengthening the hamstrings to balance them with the quadriceps is also important. When re-entering activity, proper warm-up must be stressed and a gradual increase in intensity should be followed.

Long-term prognosis

Hamstring strains that are rehabilitated fully seldom leave any lingering effects. Complete ruptures may require surgery to repair and long-term rehabilitation.

Rehabilitation exercises

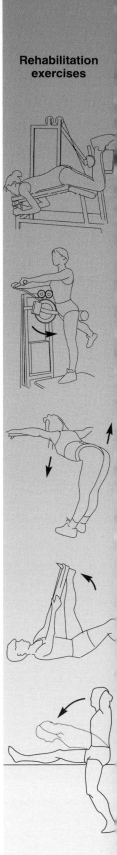

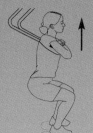

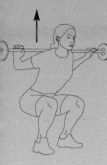

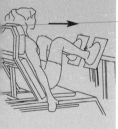

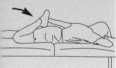

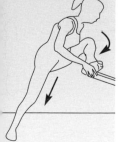

Brief outline of injury

A thigh contusion is actually a deep bruise to the muscles of the quadriceps or hamstrings near the femur. The bruising causes pain and limited flexibility in the muscle. High impact sports such as football or hockey are commonly associated with thigh bruising, but any activity that could result in falling on or getting hit in the thigh can cause a contusion.

Anatomy and physiology

The musculature of the thigh includes the *quadriceps*, comprising: *vastus lateralis, vastus medialis, vastus intermedius*, and *rectus femoris*, and the *hamstrings*, comprising: *biceps femoris, semitendinosus,* and *semimembranosus.* An impact to any of these muscles squeezes the muscle between the impacting force and the femur. This causes bleeding in the muscle near the femur. This in turn causes the formation of scar tissue that reduces muscle function. The swelling and bruising from the bleeding causes pressure on the surrounding muscle fibres reducing flexibility.

Cause of injury

Impact to the muscle from a blunt surface such as the ground, a helmet, foot, etc.

Signs and symptoms

Pain and tenderness over the injured area. Swelling and bruising may be present. Pain with weight bearing and stretching of the muscle.

Complications if left unattended

Myositis ossificans, which is characterized by the formation of bony deposits or by ossification in the muscle tissue, can develop from unattended thigh contusions. Muscle ruptures can also occur when a contusion is left untreated and activity is continued.

Immediate treatment

Rest and ice. Anti-inflammatory medication. Then heat and massage to promote blood flow and healing.

Rehabilitation and prevention

After the pain subsides it is important to regain flexibility and strength in the injured muscle. Gentle stretching will improve flexibility and help to avoid scar tissue formation. While the muscle is healing, working the surrounding muscles as tolerable may help to speed recovery by increasing blood flow and limit scarring. Use of proper protective equipment during activities and avoiding impact to the thigh will help prevent thigh contusions.

Long-term prognosis

Proper treatment of a thigh contusion will ensure that there are no future complications. Flexibility and strength should return to normal after rehabilitation of the injured muscle.

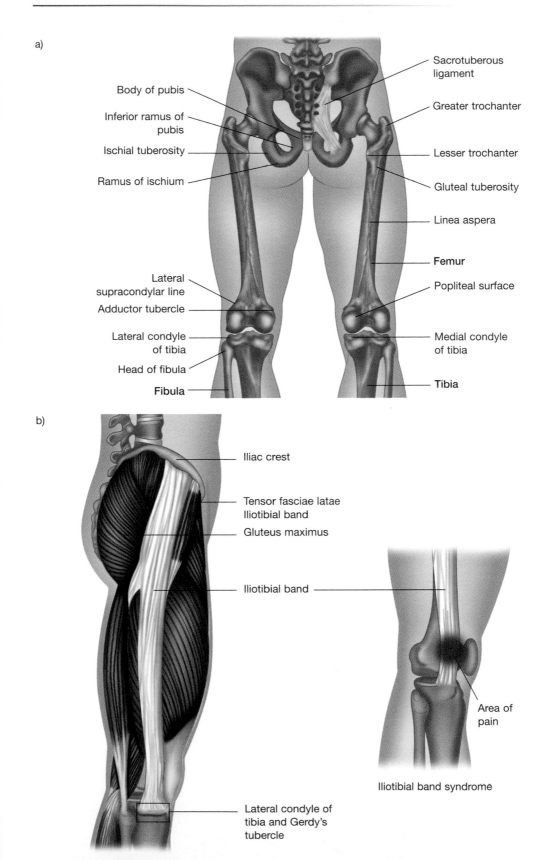

a)

Body of pubis

Inferior ramus of pubis

Ischial tuberosity

Ramus of ischium

Sacrotuberous ligament

Greater trochanter

Lesser trochanter

Gluteal tuberosity

Linea aspera

Femur

Popliteal surface

Lateral supracondylar line

Adductor tubercle

Lateral condyle of tibia

Head of fibula

Fibula

Medial condyle of tibia

Tibia

b)

Iliac crest

Tensor fasciae latae Iliotibial band

Gluteus maximus

Iliotibial band

Lateral condyle of tibia and Gerdy's tubercle

Area of pain

Iliotibial band syndrome

Figure 13.4: a) The pelvic girdle to leg, posterior view, b) anatomy of the iliotibial band.

Rehabilitation exercises

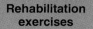

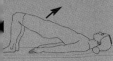

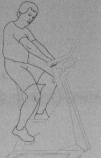

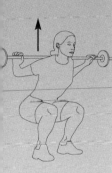

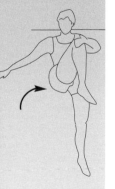

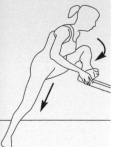

Brief outline of injury

Iliotibial band syndrome is excessive compression or friction of the iliotibial (IT) band over the greater trochanter at the hip joint, and the lateral condyle at the knee joint. This friction causes inflammation, which can be very painful whenever the knees and hips flex or extend, because it crosses over these bony prominences.

Anatomy and physiology

The iliotibial band is a non-elastic collagen cord stretching from the pelvis to below the knee. It is attached to the iliac crest at the top, blends with the tensor fasciae latae and gluteus maximus muscles, and descends down to attach to *Gerdy's tubercle* on the lateral proximal tibia. The deep fibres attach to the *linea aspera* of the femur on the lateral side of the thigh. The tensor fasciae latae flexes, abducts, and medially rotates the hip joint, and stabilizes the knee. If the iliotibial band becomes inflamed due to excessive irritation from the friction crossing over the bone, it will cause pain and tightness, possibly leading to *bursitis*.

Cause of injury

Compression or friction of the iliotibial band. Repetitive hip and knee flexion and extension while the tensor fasciae latae is contracted, such as with running. Tight tensor fasciae latae and iliotibial band. Muscle imbalances.

Signs and symptoms

Knee pain over the lateral condyle. Pain with flexion and extension of the knee.

Complications if left unattended

The iliotibial band, and accompanying tensor fasciae latae become tight due to the pain and inflammation. If left unattended this can lead to chronic pain and injuries to the knee and/or hip.

Immediate treatment

R.I.C.E.R. Anti-inflammatory medication. Then heat and massage to promote blood flow and healing.

Rehabilitation and prevention

Increasing flexibility as pain allows, will help speed recovery. After the pain has subsided, increasing strength and flexibility of all the muscles of the thighs and hips to develop balance will help prevent future issues. Identifying and fixing any errors in running form will also help to prevent recurrence of the injury.

Long-term prognosis

Iliotibial band syndrome can be treated successfully with no lingering effects. Inflammation and pain may return when the activity is resumed and form corrections must be made to prevent future problems.

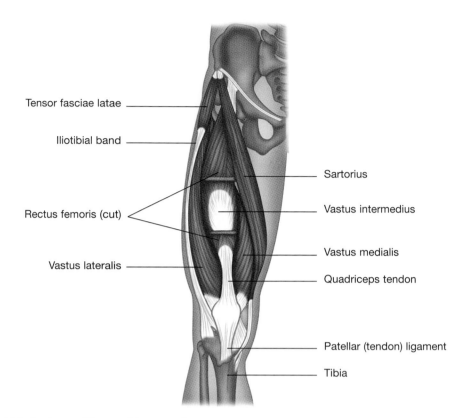

Tensor fasciae latae

Iliotibial band

Rectus femoris (cut)

Vastus lateralis

Sartorius

Vastus intermedius

Vastus medialis

Quadriceps tendon

Patellar (tendon) ligament

Tibia

Figure 13.5: Anatomy of the quadriceps tendon.

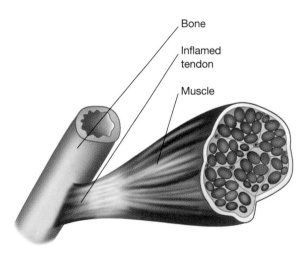

Bone

Inflamed tendon

Muscle

Quadriceps tendinitis

Rehabilitation exercises

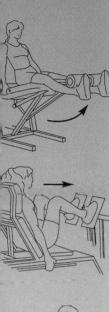

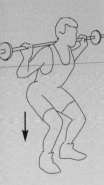

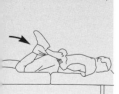

Brief outline of injury

Quadriceps tendinitis, like other versions of tendinitis, involves inflammation of the tendon. This can be a result of repetitive stresses to the quadriceps, or excessive stress before the muscle is conditioned. Pain just above the patella (knee cap), especially when extending the knee, usually accompanies this injury.

Anatomy and physiology

The quadriceps tendon attaches to, and covers the patella, becoming the *patellar (tendon) ligament* below this and attaching to the tibia. The patella runs in the groove of the femur as the knee flexes and extends, which results in the tendon passing over this bone as well. Repetitive stress can cause inflammation of the tendon, especially under contraction, such as when accelerating or decelerating. Minor tears may also occur in the tendon as well when the stress is too much for the tendon to handle.

Cause of injury

Repetitive stress to the tendon, e.g. running or jumping. Repetitive acceleration and deceleration, e.g. hurdling or football. Untreated injury to the quadriceps.

Signs and symptoms

Pain just above the patella. Jumping, running, kneeling, or walking down stairs may aggravate the pain.

Complications if left unattended

The quadriceps muscles may become inflamed, and the tendon will become weak if left untreated. This could lead to a rupture of the tendon. A change in gait or landing form can lead to other injuries as well.

Immediate treatment

Rest and ice. Anti-inflammatory medication. Training modification.

Rehabilitation and prevention

Rehabilitation should include stretching and strengthening exercises for the quadriceps. Activities such as swimming can be helpful to reduce the stress on the tendon during rehabilitation. Return to a normal activity schedule should be delayed until pain subsides completely and strength is restored. Keeping the quadriceps flexible and strong will help prevent this condition.

Long-term prognosis

A full recovery with no long-term disability or lingering effects can be expected in most cases of tendinitis, and surgery is only necessary in extremely rare cases.

Chapter

14

Sports Injuries of the
Knee

Acute

080: Medial Collateral Ligament Sprain

081: Anterior Cruciate Ligament Sprain

082: Meniscus Tear

Chronic

083: Bursitis

084: Knee (Synovial) Plica

085: Osgood-Schlatter Syndrome

086: Osteochondritis Dissecans

087: Patellofemoral Pain Syndrome

088: Patellar Tendinitis (Jumper's Knee)

089: Chondromalacia Patellae (Runner's Knee)

090: Subluxing Knee Cap

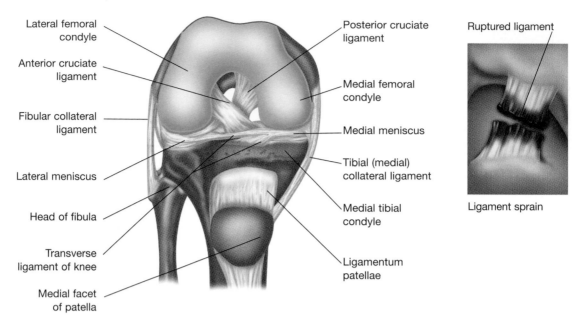

Lateral femoral condyle

Anterior cruciate ligament

Fibular collateral ligament

Lateral meniscus

Head of fibula

Transverse ligament of knee

Medial facet of patella

Posterior cruciate ligament

Medial femoral condyle

Medial meniscus

Tibial (medial) collateral ligament

Medial tibial condyle

Ligamentum patellae

Ruptured ligament

Ligament sprain

Figure 14.1: The knee joint, right leg, anterior view.

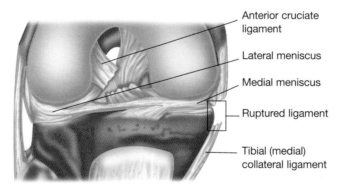

Anterior cruciate ligament

Lateral meniscus

Medial meniscus

Ruptured ligament

Tibial (medial) collateral ligament

Meniscus tear

Rehabilitation exercises

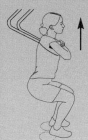

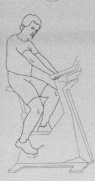

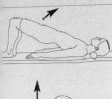

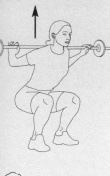

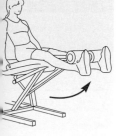

Brief outline of injury

A ligament is tough, fibrous connective tissue that connects bone to bone, and provides support and strength to a joint. Medial collateral ligament sprain involves tearing or stretching of this ligament, and is usually caused by force applied to the outside of the knee joint as in a tackle in football.

Anatomy and physiology

The medial (tibial) collateral ligament is one of the four supporting ligaments of the knee. It is a broad, flat band about 12 cm long, and spans the joint on the inside of the knee running from the *medial epicondyle* of the femur to the *medial condyle* of the tibial shaft. Some fibres are fused to the *medial meniscus*. This ligament is designed to hold the knee joint together on the medial (inside) surface. Force applied to the outside of the knee causes the inside of the knee to open, stretching the medial collateral ligament. The extent of the stretch determines whether the ligament simply stretches, tears partially, or completely tears.

Cause of injury

Force applied to the outside of the knee joint.

Signs and symptoms

Pain over the medial portion of the knee. Swelling and tenderness. Instability in the knee and pain with weight bearing.

Complications if left unattended

The ligament, in rare cases, may repair itself if left unattended but could lead to a more severe sprain. The pain and instability in the knee may not go away. Continued activity on the injured knee could lead to injuries in the other ligaments, due to the instability.

Immediate treatment

R.I.C.E.R. Immobilization. Anti-inflammatory medication.

Rehabilitation and prevention

Depending on the severity of the sprain, simple rest and gradual introduction back into activity may be enough. For more severe sprains, braces may be needed during the strengthening phase of rehabilitation and the early portion of the return to activity. The most severe sprains may require extended immobilization and rest from the activity. As range of motion and strength begins to return, stationary bikes and other equipment may be used to ease back into activity. Ensuring adequate strength in the thigh muscles and conditioning before starting any activity that is susceptible to hits to the knee will help prevent these types of injuries.

Long-term prognosis

The ligament will usually heal with no limitations, although in some cases there is residual *looseness* in the medial part of the knee. Very rarely, surgery is required to repair the ligaments. Meniscus tearing may also result from a sprain that may require surgical repair.

Brief outline of injury

The anterior cruciate ligament (ACL) is one of the four ligaments of the knee and it holds the knee together from the front. It is commonly injured in sports where there are a lot of direction changes and possible impacts. Football, lacrosse, and other fast moving games that require quick changes often result in ACL sprains. The most common mechanism for this injury is when the knee rotates while the foot is planted. Sharp pain at the time of the injury accompanied by swelling in the knee joint may be a sign of an ACL tear.

Anatomy and physiology

The anterior cruciate ligament extends obliquely upwards, laterally and backwards from the *anterior intercondylar area* of the tibia to the medial surface of the *lateral femoral condyle*. This ligament prevents posterior displacement of the femur on the tibia, and also helps check hyperextension of the knee. When the foot is planted fixing the tibia in place, and the knee is rotated forcefully, the stress can cause a tear in the ACL. This can range from minor tearing of a few fibres to a complete tear. It can also be torn as the result of a hard blow to the knee; usually other ligaments and the meniscus are involved as well.

Cause of injury

Forceful twisting of the knee when the foot is planted. Occasionally a forceful blow to the knee, especially if the foot is fixed as well.

Signs and symptoms

Pain immediately that may go away. Swelling in the knee joint. Instability in the knee, especially with the tibia.

Complications if left unattended

If left unattended, this injury may not heal properly. The instability in the joint could lead to injury to other ligaments. Chronic pain and instability could lead to future limitations.

Immediate treatment

R.I.C.E.R. (immediate referral to a sports medicine professional). Immobilization.

Rehabilitation and prevention

Once stability and strength return and pain subsides, gradual introduction of activities such as stationary biking can be undertaken. Range of motion and strengthening exercises are an important part of rehabilitation. Swimming and other non-weight bearing exercises may be used until the strength returns to normal. Strengthening the muscles of the quadriceps, hamstrings, and calves will help to protect the anterior cruciate ligament. Proper conditioning before beginning high impact activities will also provide protection.

Long-term prognosis

ACL sprains that involve a complete tear often require surgery to reattach the ligament. Minor sprains can often be healed completely without surgery. Return to full activity may be a prolonged process and some activities may be limited.

Rehabilitation exercises

**Rehabilitation
exercises**

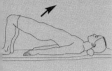

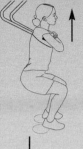

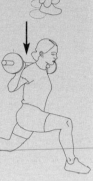

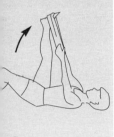

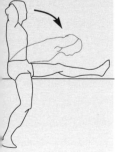

Brief outline of injury

The menisci are discs of fibrocartilage that cushion the knee joint. Tearing of the menisci can occur with forceful twisting of the knee, or may accompany other injuries such as ligament sprains. The *unhappy triad* is when a blow to the lateral side of the knee causes tearing of the medial collateral ligament, the anterior cruciate ligament, and the menisci.

Anatomy and physiology

The menisci is actually composed of two parts, the *medial* and *lateral meniscus*. The medial meniscus rests on the medial plateau of the tibia and the lateral meniscus rests on the lateral plateau. Each meniscus is C-shaped and provides cushioning and protection for the ends of the femur and tibia, acting as a shock absorber. The menisci help to distribute the weight evenly through the joint. Forceful twisting of the knee, especially if bent, can cause tearing of the menisci. This is often seen in sports that require a planting of the foot to quickly change direction. The medial meniscus is injured much more frequently than the lateral meniscus, mainly due to it being more securely attached to the tibia, and, therefore, less mobile.

Cause of injury

Forceful twisting of the knee joint, most commonly seen when the knee is also bent. May accompany ligament strains as well.

Signs and symptoms

Pain in the knee joint. Some swelling may be noted. Catching, or locking, in the joint.

Complications if left unattended

The loose bodies and jagged edges of a meniscal tear can cause premature wear on the cartilage at the ends of the bones and under the patella. This can lead to arthritic conditions and a fluid build-up in the knee joint.

Immediate treatment

R.I.C.E.R. Anti-inflammatory medication.

Rehabilitation and prevention

After repair of a meniscal tear, it is important to strengthen the muscles surrounding the knee to prevent the injury from happening again. Strong quadriceps and hamstrings help support the knee and prevent the twisting that might cause a tear. The muscles should be stretched regularly as well since tight muscles can also cause problems in the knee. After repair of a meniscus tear, weight bearing should be encouraged as tolerable, but as with any restart of activity it should be done gradually.

Long-term prognosis

A tear to a meniscus usually requires arthroscopic surgery to repair. The surgery requires removal of the torn edges of the meniscus but leaves the main body of the meniscus intact. Therefore, most meniscus tears heal fully with no long-term limitations.

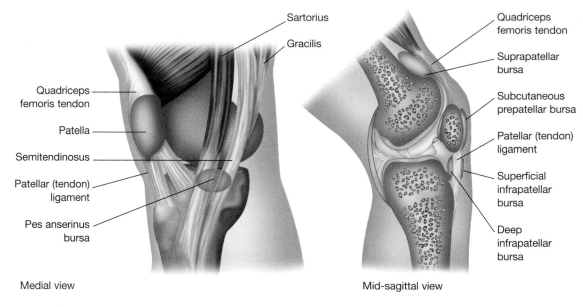

Sartorius

Gracilis

Quadriceps femoris tendon

Patella

Semitendinosus

Patellar (tendon) ligament

Pes anserinus bursa

Quadriceps femoris tendon

Suprapatellar bursa

Subcutaneous prepatellar bursa

Patellar (tendon) ligament

Superficial infrapatellar bursa

Deep infrapatellar bursa

Medial view

Mid-sagittal view

Figure 14.2: The knee joint.

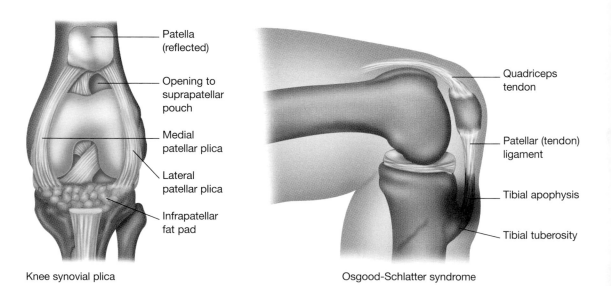

Patella (reflected)

Opening to suprapatellar pouch

Medial patellar plica

Lateral patellar plica

Infrapatellar fat pad

Quadriceps tendon

Patellar (tendon) ligament

Tibial apophysis

Tibial tuberosity

Knee synovial plica

Osgood-Schlatter syndrome

083: BURSITIS

Rehabilitation exercises

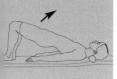

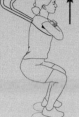

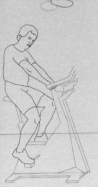

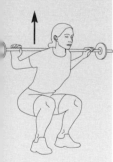

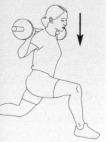

Brief outline of injury

Bursitis can be a painful condition, especially when located in the weight bearing knee joint. Since the job of the bursa is to cushion and lubricate the joint where friction is likely to occur, inflammation will result in pain in most weight bearing, flexion, or extension activities. The knee joint has on average fourteen bursae.

Anatomy and physiology

A bursa is a sac filled with a viscid fluid. The deep bursa formed by the joint capsule at the knee, the *suprapatellar bursa*, is the largest bursa in the body. It is located between the femur and quadriceps femoris tendon. Three other major bursae of the knee are the *subcutaneous prepatellar bursa*, located between the skin and the anterior surface of the patella, the *superficial infrapatellar bursa*, located between the skin and the patellar (tendon) ligament, and the *deep infrapatellar bursa*, located between the tibial tuberosity and the patellar (tendon) ligament. Finally, the *pes anserinus bursa* is located at the lower inside of the knee joint where *sartorius, gracilis*, and *semitendinosus* insert as the conjoined *pes anserinus tendon*. The prepatellar bursa is the most commonly injured due to its superficial location. Repetitive kneeling or impact to the knee cap can damage this bursa. The infrapatellar bursae are most commonly inflamed during jumping and landing from repetitive friction of the patellar (tendon) ligament. The pes anserinus bursa is less commonly involved in injuries but can result from load bearing on the inside of the knee, as seen with improper gait or use of worn or improperly sized running shoes.

Cause of injury

Repetitive pressure or trauma to the bursa. Repetitive friction between the bursa and tendon or bone.

Signs and symptoms

Pain and tenderness. Mild swelling, due to release of the fluid in the bursal sac. Pain and stiffness when kneeling or walking downstairs.

Complications if left unattended

If a bursa is allowed to rupture and release its fluid, the natural cushioning will be lost. The build-up of fluid will cause loss of mobility in the joint as well.

Immediate treatment

R.I.C.E.R. Anti-inflammatory medication.

Rehabilitation and prevention

Strengthening the muscles around the knee will help to support the joint, and increasing flexibility also will relieve some of the pressure exerted by the tendons upon the bursa. Frequent rests when required to be in a kneeling or crouching position also help to prevent this condition. Identifying any underlying problems, such as improper equipment or form is important during rehabilitation to prevent it from recurring.

Long-term prognosis

Bursitis is seldom a long-term concern if treated properly. Occasionally draining of the fluid from the joint is necessary.

SPORTS INJURIES OF THE KNEE

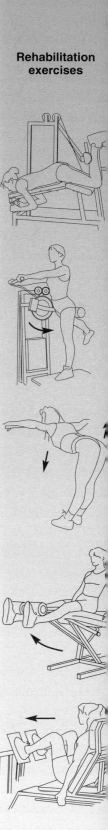

Rehabilitation exercises

Brief outline of injury

The synovial plica is a thin fibrous membrane that is a remnant from the foetal knee development. The plica once divided the knee into three separate compartments during foetal development but then became a part of the knee structure as the compartments became one protective cavity. The plica may become inflamed due to friction or pinching between the patella and the femur. This is common when the knee is flexed and placed under a stress.

Anatomy and physiology

When a foetus is developing, the knee is divided into three compartments. As the foetus reaches full development these three compartments become one large protective cavity, the *synovial membrane*. Most people have some remnant of these divisions, the plica, left over as thin membranes. They are usually located on the medial side of the knee, and extend from the suprapatellar fossa along the medial patellar border. These *plica* seldom cause problems by themselves. When friction or a pinching between the femur and patella occur, the synovial plica may become inflamed causing it to thicken, which in turn causes more friction creating a vicious cycle.

Cause of injury

Trauma to the flexed knee. Repetitive stress, especially with medial weight bearing, e.g. biking.

Signs and symptoms

Pain. Tenderness over the synovial plica.

Complications if left unattended

The synovial plica will continue to become inflamed and limit flexion activity in the knee if left unattended. The pain may also cause a change in gait or running form that could lead to other overuse injuries.

Immediate treatment

Reducing activity. R.I.C.E.R. Anti-inflammatory medication.

Rehabilitation and prevention

Strengthening the quadriceps and hamstrings will take pressure off the synovial plica. Increasing flexibility in these muscles will also relieve pressure that may be irritating the condition. Use of proper equipment, especially running shoes, can eliminate the irritation and force the knee back into proper alignment during activity.

Long-term prognosis

Once pain subsides, a return to normal activity can be expected. Very rarely is arthroscopic surgery required to remove the plica. No adverse effects have been found from the removal of the synovial plica and a complete return to activity can be expected.

SPORTS INJURIES OF THE KNEE

Rehabilitation exercises

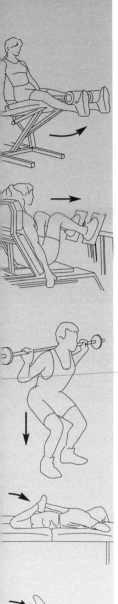

Brief outline of injury

Osgood-Schlatter syndrome is a traction-type injury of the tibial apophysis, where the patellar (tendon) ligament pulls on the tibial tuberosity just below the knee. It is a condition that affects active young teens, and is more prevalent in males (particularly boys aged 10–15) than females, and has a slightly higher prevalence in the left knee than the right. When the quadriceps are tight, or there is repetitive flexion and extension, this stress may cause inflammation and pain. A similar condition, *Larsen-Johansson syndrome*, results in pain and tenderness over the inferior pole (extremity) of the patella, but is treated in a similar way to Osgood-Schlatter syndrome.

Anatomy and physiology

The patellar (tendon) ligament attaches to the patella and then continues down to attach below the knee joint at the *tibial tuberosity*. The bones of a developing skeleton are not as hard as mature bones. So the force of the ligament pulling up on the tibia may cause small avulsion fractures, leading to inflammation and pain. The body may try to repair and protect this area by building more bone, resulting in a bony prominence just under the knee, which gives the characteristic tibial bump. This is exacerbated in adolescents by a growth spurt, since the lengthening of bones often exceeds the growth of the muscles attached, causing tight muscles. This puts additional force on the attached tendons. During running, jumping and kicking activities, the quadriceps must contract and relax continuously, which also stresses the attachment at the tibia.

Cause of injury

Tight quadriceps due to growth spurt. Prior knee injury. Repetitive contractions of the quadriceps muscle.

Signs and symptoms

Pain, worse at full extension and during squatting, subsides with rest. Swelling over the tibial tuberosity, just under the knee. Redness and inflammation of the skin just below the knee.

Complications if left unattended

If left unattended the condition will continue to cause pain and inflammation and could lead to muscle loss in the quadriceps. In rare cases, untreated Osgood-Schlatter syndrome could lead to a complete avulsion fracture of the tibia.

Immediate treatment

R.I.C.E.R. Anti-inflammatory medication.

Rehabilitation and prevention

Most cases of Osgood-Schlatter syndrome respond well to rest and then a regimen of stretching and strengthening the quadriceps muscles. Limiting activities that cause pain and tend to aggravate the issue is important during recovery. Gradual increases in intensity and proper warm-up techniques will help prevent this condition.

Long-term prognosis

This condition tends to correct itself as the bone becomes stronger and mature. The pain and inflammation go away and there are seldom any long-term effects. Rare cases may require corticosteroid injections to aid recovery.

a)

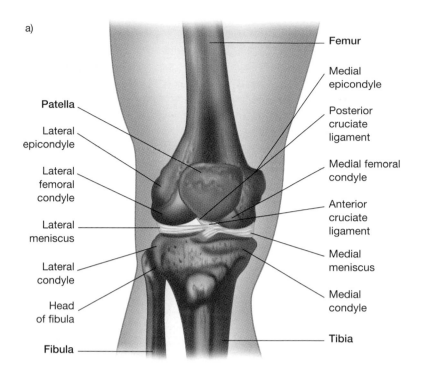

Femur

Patella

Lateral epicondyle

Lateral femoral condyle

Lateral meniscus

Lateral condyle

Head of fibula

Fibula

Medial epicondyle

Posterior cruciate ligament

Medial femoral condyle

Anterior cruciate ligament

Medial meniscus

Medial condyle

Tibia

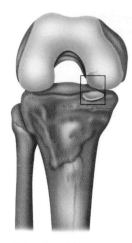

Osteochondritis dissecans

b)

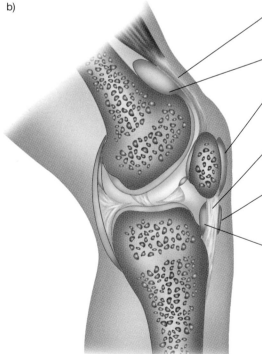

Quadriceps femoris tendon

Suprapatellar bursa

Subcutaneous prepatellar bursa

Patellar (tendon) ligament

Superficial infrapatellar bursa

Deep infrapatellar bursa

Figure 14.3: The knee joint, a) anterior view, b) mid-sagittal view.

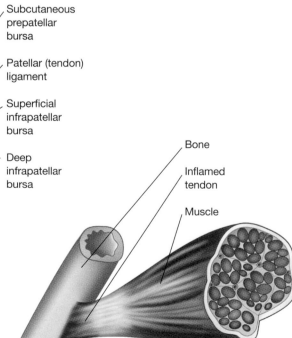

Bone

Inflamed tendon

Muscle

Patellar tendinitis

086: OSTEOCHONDRITIS DISSECANS

Rehabilitation exercises

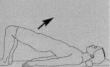

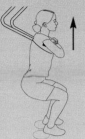

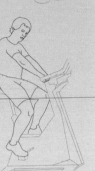

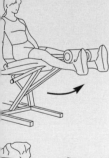

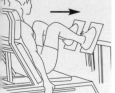

Brief outline of injury

Osteochondritis dissecans (loose bodies in the joint) occurs when a fragment of bone adjacent to the articular surface of a joint is deprived of its blood supply, leading to *avascular necrosis*. This causes the cartilage to become brittle and a piece, or pieces, may break off. If the cartilage gets into the joint, it can cause pain and inflammation. Although found in several joints, this condition is most commonly associated with the knee and is particularly prevalent in males aged 10–20 years.

Anatomy and physiology

The bones are covered by cartilage at their ends. This cartilage protects the bones from excessive wear. If the blood supply to this area is lost due to a prior injury or other condition, the cartilage becomes hard and brittle. Impact or repetitive wear may cause it to break. If the broken pieces stay attached to the bone, there is generally no problem. When they release into the joint, the feeling of instability and a "clicking" or locking in the joint may be noticed. This causes premature wear in the joint.

Cause of injury

Loss of blood supply to the end of the bone and attached cartilage. Impact to the joint causing a tearing or breaking of the cartilage at the bone end. Repetitive friction leading to the cartilage becoming brittle and breaking away.

Signs and symptoms

Aching, diffuse pain, and swelling, especially during activity. Stiffness with rest. Clicking, or weakness in the joint. Momentary locking if the bony fragment has displaced and is free floating within the joint.

Complications if left unattended

If left unattended, the loose bodies will continue to cause damage to the inner surface of the joint and could eventually lead to degenerative osteoarthritis. The loose bodies could also lead to tearing or "grooving" of other cartilage in the joint.

Immediate treatment

Rest and referral to a sports medicine professional. Immobilization. Anti-inflammatory medication. Positive diagnosis made with a radiograph.

Rehabilitation and prevention

Strengthening the muscles surrounding the affected joint will help support it better during activity. Limiting the amount of time spent doing repetitive movement with the joint may also be required. Treatment of minor injuries to the joint may also help stop the chance of the blood supply being cut off. Limit activities that cause pain and gradually work back into a full schedule.

Long-term prognosis

If the broken cartilage does not release from the bone, it may repair itself. However, if it becomes lodged in the joint and the body does not dissolve it, surgery may be required. In younger athletes, a complete recovery and return to activity may be expected. In older athletes, the development of degenerative osteoarthritis is usually a by-product of this condition.

087: PATELLOFEMORAL PAIN SYNDROME

Rehabilitation exercises

Brief outline of injury

Pain in the patella (knee cap), especially after sitting for a long time or running downhill, may be a result of a fairly common condition called *patellofemoral pain syndrome*. The pain may result from incorrect movement of the patella over the femur, or tight tendons. The articular cartilage under the knee cap may become inflamed as well, leading to another condition called *chondromalacia patellae*. Found more commonly in women.

Anatomy and physiology

The patella is a small triangular sesamoid bone within the tendon of the quadriceps femoris muscle and forms the front of the knee joint. It is attached above to the quadriceps tendon, and below to the patellar (tendon) ligament, and articulates with the *patellofemoral groove* between the *femoral condyles* to form the *patellofemoral joint*. The angle formed between the two lines of pull of the quadriceps muscle and the patellar (tendon) ligament is known as the *Q-angle*. If the patella moves out of its normal path, even slightly, it can cause irritation and pain. Tight tendons also place pressure on the patella causing inflammation.

Cause of injury

Incorrect running form or improper shoes. Weak or tight quadriceps. Chronic patella dislocations.

Signs and symptoms

Pain on and under the knee cap, and worsens after sitting for extended periods or walking downstairs. Clicking or grinding may be felt when flexing the knee. Dull, aching pain in the center of the knee.

Complications if left unattended

The inflammation from this condition if left unattended can worsen and cause more permanent damage to the surrounding structures. If the tendon becomes inflamed, it could eventually rupture. The cartilage under the patella may also become inflamed.

Immediate treatment

Rest, which can be simply reducing the intensity and duration. Ice and anti-inflammatory medication.

Rehabilitation and prevention

Rehabilitation starts with restoring the strength and flexibility of the quadriceps. When returning to activity after pain has subsided, gradual increases in intensity, limiting repetitive stresses on the knee and proper warm-up techniques will ensure that the pain does not return.

Strong, flexible quadriceps and hamstrings and avoiding overuse will help prevent patellofemoral pain syndrome. A good warm-up before training will also help.

Long-term prognosis

With complete treatment there are seldom any long lasting effects. If the condition does not respond to treatment, surgical intervention may be necessary.

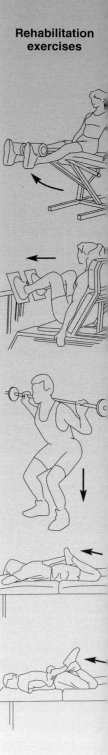

088: PATELLAR TENDINITIS (JUMPER'S KNEE)

Rehabilitation exercises

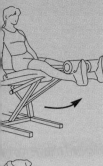

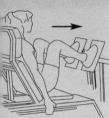

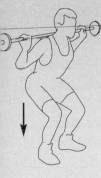

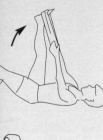

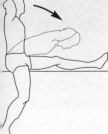

Brief outline of injury

Activities that require repetitive jumping like basketball or volleyball can lead to tendinitis in the patellar (tendon) ligament, also referred to as *jumper's knee*. The force placed on the tendon over time can lead to inflammation and pain. The pain is generally felt just below the knee cap.

Anatomy and physiology

Patellar tendinitis affects the teno-osseous junctions of the quadriceps tendon as it attaches to the superior pole (extremity) of the patella, and the patellar (tendon) ligament as it attaches to the inferior pole of the patella and the tibial tuberosity. Pain is concentrated on the patellar (tendon) ligament, but can also occur at the insertion of the patellar (tendon) ligament into the *tibial tuberosity*. The patellar (tendon) ligament is involved in extending the lower leg, but is also the first area to experience shock when landing from a jump. It is forced to stretch as the quadriceps contracts to slow down the flexion of the knee. This repetitive stress can lead to minor trauma in the tendon, which will lead to inflammation. Repetitive flexing and extending of the knee also places stress on this tendon if the tendon does not travel in the required path.

Cause of injury

Repetitive jumping and landing activities. Running and kicking activities. Untreated minor injury to the patellar tendon.

Signs and symptoms

Pain and inflammation of the patellar tendon, especially from repetitive or eccentric knee extension activity or kneeling. Swelling and tenderness around the tendon.

Complications if left unattended

As with most tendinitis, inflammation that is left untreated will cause additional irritation, which causes more inflammation, setting up a vicious cycle. This can eventually lead to a rupture of the tendon. Damage to surrounding tissue may also occur.

Immediate treatment

R.I.C.E.R. Anti-inflammatory medication.

Rehabilitation and prevention

Stretching the quadriceps, hamstrings and calves will help relieve pressure on the patellar tendon. During rehabilitation it is important to identify the conditions that caused the injury in the first place. Thorough warm-up and proper conditioning can help prevent the onset of this condition. A support strap placed below the knee may be needed at first to support the tendon during the initial return to activity. Prevention of this condition requires strong quadriceps and a good strength balance between the muscles that surround the knee.

Long-term prognosis

Complete recovery without lingering effects can be expected with good treatment. Occasionally, it may return due to a weakened tendon, especially in older athletes.

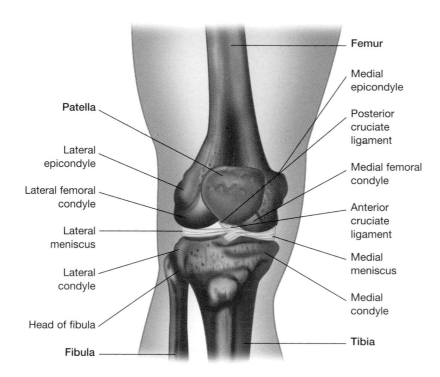

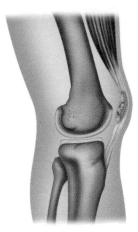

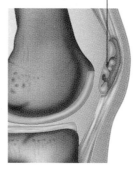

Chondromalacia patellae

Figure 14.4: The knee joint, anterior view.

Chondromalacia patellae

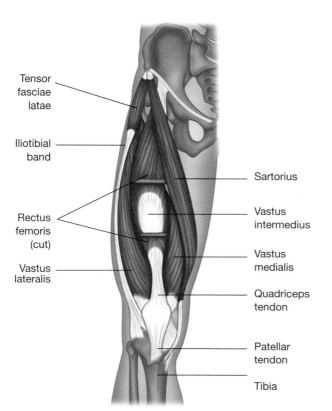

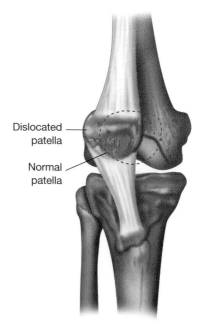

Figure 14.5: The quadriceps.

Subluxing knee cap

089: CHONDROMALACIA PATELLAE (RUNNER'S KNEE)

Rehabilitation exercises

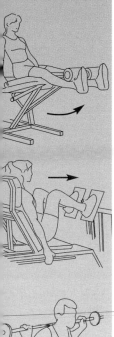

Brief outline of injury

Softening and degeneration of the articular cartilage of the patella (knee cap) in athletes is usually a result of overuse, trauma, or abnormal forces on the knee. In older adults it can be a result of degenerative arthritis. Pain under the knee cap and a grating sensation when the knee is extended are possible signs of this condition.

Anatomy and physiology

The underside of the patella is protected by *articular (hyaline) cartilage*, which is made up of collagen fibres and water. The cartilage can become damaged and softened by repetitive micro-trauma due to overuse or abnormal load bearing on the knee. This degeneration makes the surface rough instead of its usual smooth surface, which causes additional inflammation and pain. Generally described in four progressive stages, from softening and blistering, to full cartilage defects and subchondrial bone exposure.

Cause of injury

Repetitive micro-trauma to the cartilage through overuse conditions. Misalignment of the knee cap. Previous fracture or dislocation of the knee cap.

Signs and symptoms

Pain that worsens after sitting for prolonged periods or when using stairs or rising from a seated position. Tenderness over the knee cap. Grating or grinding sensation when the knee is extended.

Complications if left unattended

Cartilage that degenerates and becomes rough can cause scarring in the bone surface it rubs against. This in turn causes more inflammation. Cartilage can also be torn when it is rough leading to loose bodies in the joint.

Immediate treatment

Rest and ice. Anti-inflammatory medication.

Rehabilitation and prevention

Limiting activity until the pain subsides and gradually re-entering the activity is important. Strengthening and stretching the quadriceps is important to relieve pressure on the patella. Activities that increase the pain, such as deep knee bending, should be avoided until completely pain free. Avoid abnormal stress on the knee, and keep the hamstrings and quadriceps strong and flexible to prevent this condition.

Long-term prognosis

Chondromalacia patellae commonly responds well to therapy and anti-inflammatory medication. In rare cases, surgery may be required to correct a misalignment in the knee cap.

090: SUBLUXING KNEE CAP

Brief outline of injury

A subluxation or dislocation of the knee cap (patella) commonly occurs during deceleration. The knee cap slides partially out of the groove that is designed for it but does not limit mobility. Pain and swelling may accompany this condition. Athletes who have a muscle imbalance or a structural deformity, such as a high knee cap, have a higher chance of a subluxing knee cap.

Anatomy and physiology

The patella is a small triangular sesamoid bone within the tendon of the quadriceps femoris muscle and forms the front of the knee joint. It is attached above to the quadriceps tendon, and below to the patellar (tendon) ligament, and articulates with the *patellofemoral groove* between the *femoral condyles* to form the *patellofemoral joint*. The patella slides over the groove when the knee flexes. If the outer muscle of the quadriceps, the *vastus lateralis*, is stronger than the inner muscle, the *vastus medialis*, this imbalance may cause an uneven pull on the knee cap forcing it out of the normal groove. In addition, the lateral femoral condyle and medial patellar bone may be bruised. This happens with forceful contractions such as planting, changing direction, or landing from a jump.

Cause of injury

Strength imbalance between the outer quadriceps group and the inner group. Impact to the side of the knee cap. Twisting of the knee.

Signs and symptoms

Feeling of pressure under the knee cap. Pain and swelling behind the knee cap. Pain when bending or straightening the knee.

Complications if left unattended

Continued subluxations can cause small fractures in the patella, cartilage tears, and stress on the tendons. Failure to treat a subluxation could lead to chronic subluxations.

Immediate treatment

R.I.C.E.R. Anti-inflammatory medication.

Rehabilitation and prevention

During rehabilitation, activities that do not aggravate the injury should be sought, such as swimming or biking instead of running. Strengthening of the vastus medialis and stretching the vastus lateralis will help correct the muscle imbalance that may cause this condition. A brace to hold the knee cap in place may be needed when initially returning to activity. To prevent subluxations, it is important to keep the muscles surrounding the knee strong and flexible and avoid impact to the knee cap.

Long-term prognosis

Subluxations respond well to rest, rehabilitation, and anti-inflammatory measures. Rarely surgery may be required to prevent recurring subluxations due to misalignment or loose support structures.

Chapter
15

Sports Injuries of the
Lower Leg

Acute

091: Fractures (Tibia, Fibula)

092: Calf Strain

093: Achilles Tendon Strain

Chronic

094: Achilles Tendinitis

095: Medial Tibial Pain Syndrome (Shin Splints)

096: Stress Fracture

097: Anterior Compartment Syndrome

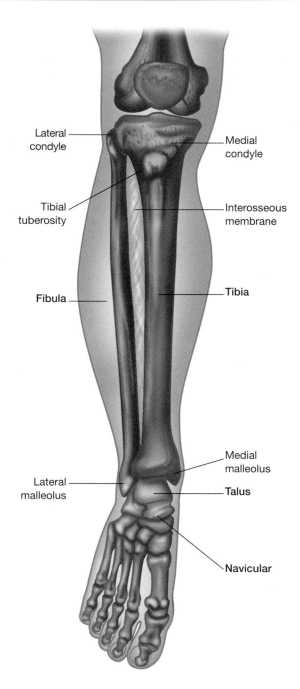

Lateral condyle

Medial condyle

Tibial tuberosity

Interosseous membrane

Fibula

Tibia

Medial malleolus

Lateral malleolus

Talus

Navicular

Figure 15.1: Tibia and fibula of the right leg, anterior view.

Rehabilitation exercises

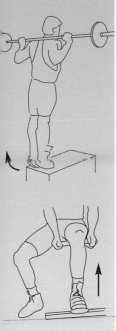

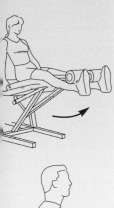

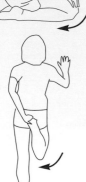

Brief outline of injury

Most human bones have outer shells of *cortical bone*, which means that the porosity is low, with *cancellous bone* underneath (high porosity). The cortical bone means that the structure is stiffer and capable of withstanding great stress. When the outer shell is cracked it is called a *fracture*. The bone may be either partially fractured or completely broken.

Anatomy and physiology

The tibia *(shin bone)* is the larger and more medial of the bones in the lower leg. At the proximal end, the *medial* and *lateral condyles* articulate with the distal end of the femur to form the knee joint. The *tibial tuberosity* is a roughened area on the anterior surface of the tibia. The fibula lies lateral and parallel to the tibia and is thin and sticklike. The fibula is not a weight bearing bone and plays no part in the knee joint, the tibia is the only weight bearing bone of the lower leg. Both bones meet at the ankle. Although either bone can be fractured alone, they are most commonly fractured together. Most fractures involve the proximal (near the knee), or distal (near the ankle) ends of the bone. Due to the thin covering of skin and other tissue over the tibia, these fractures are often *open fractures*, meaning the broken bone ends break the skin.

Cause of injury

Direct force (impact) to the bones along the shaft or extreme loading of the bone, such as with a landing from a high fall. Rotational or indirect forces on the bones, e.g. tackle in football. Twisting, especially when the bone is under a load or when the foot is fixed.

Signs and symptoms

Pain, inability to walk or bear weight, and often inability to move the leg. Deformity may be present at the fracture site, or the fracture may be open (see above). Swelling and tenderness.

Complications if left unattended

Instability in the lower leg is one long-term complication of an untreated fracture. Blood vessel damage from a fracture can lead to internal bleeding and swelling as well as circulation problems for the foot. Nerve involvement can lead to serious problems such as *drop foot* or a loss of sensation in the lower leg and foot.

Immediate treatment

Immobilize the leg. Control any bleeding that might be present with an open fracture. Seek medical attention immediately.

Rehabilitation and prevention

After the fracture has healed, it will be necessary to rebuild the strength and flexibility of the muscles in the lower leg. Range of motion activities may be needed for the knee and ankle depending on the location of the fracture and the extent of immobilization required. When the fracture has healed a gradual re-entry into activity must be observed to prevent re-injury. Strong calf and anterior tibialis muscles will help protect the tibia and fibula.

Long-term prognosis

If set properly and allowed to heal fully, a fracture should not present any future problems. In some cases a rod or pins may be needed to hold the bones in place during healing. Surgery may be required in a few cases where blood vessel or nerve damage is severe.

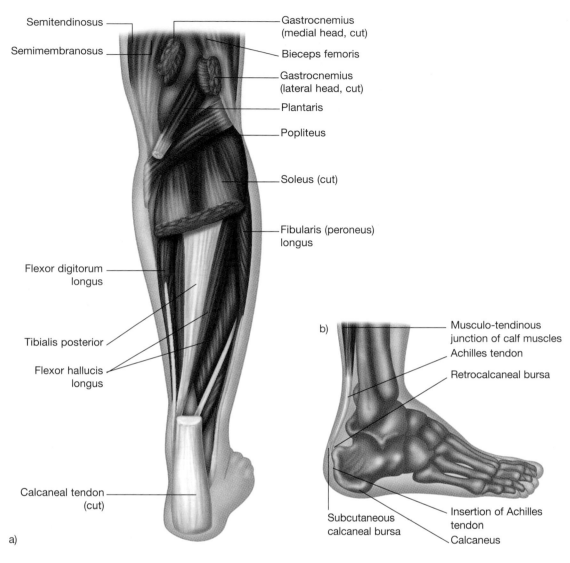

Semitendinosus

Semimembranosus

Gastrocnemius
(medial head, cut)

Bieceps femoris

Gastrocnemius
(lateral head, cut)

Plantaris

Popliteus

Soleus (cut)

Fibularis (peroneus)
longus

Flexor digitorum
longus

Tibialis posterior

Flexor hallucis
longus

Calcaneal tendon
(cut)

a)

b)

Musculo-tendinous
junction of calf muscles

Achilles tendon

Retrocalcaneal bursa

Subcutaneous
calcaneal bursa

Insertion of Achilles
tendon

Calcaneus

Figure 15.2: a) The calf muscles, right leg, posterior view, b) Achilles tendon.

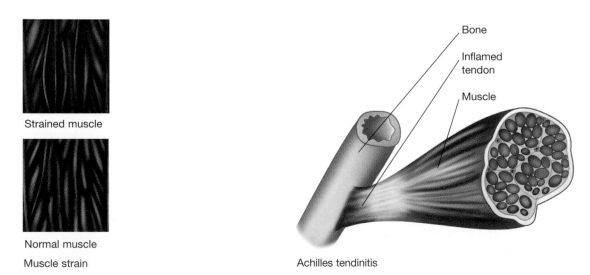

Strained muscle

Normal muscle

Muscle strain

Bone

Inflamed
tendon

Muscle

Achilles tendinitis

Rehabilitation exercises

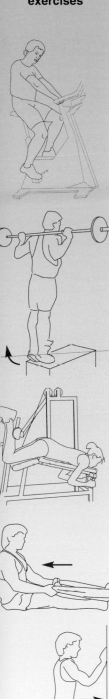

Brief outline of injury

Failing to warm-up properly can lead to muscle strains. The calf muscles are used when taking off during a sprint, when jumping, changing directions, or when coming out of the bottom of a deep squat. These are usually explosive movements requiring forceful contractions of the calf muscles, which can lead to a muscle strain. Strains can result from incorrect foot positioning during an activity or an eccentric contraction beyond the strength level of the muscle.

Anatomy and physiology

The muscles of the calf include the gastrocnemius, plantaris, and soleus, known as the *triceps surae*. These muscles attach to the foot through the *Achilles tendon*. The *popliteal fossa* at the back of the knee is formed inferiorly by the bellies of gastrocnemius and plantaris, laterally by the tendon of biceps femoris, and medially by the tendons of semimembranosus and semitendinosus. The calf muscles are responsible for extending the foot, and rising up on the toes. When taking off or changing direction, the calf muscle must contract forcefully. This contraction can cause tearing of the muscle at the attachment of the tendon. An eccentric contraction, a contraction while the muscle stretches, such as when landing from a jump, can also cause a tear if the muscle is fatigued or not strong enough to handle it.

Cause of injury

Forceful contraction of the gastrocnemius or soleus muscle. Forceful eccentric contraction. Improper foot position when pushing off or landing.

Signs and symptoms

Pain in the calf muscle, usually mid-calf. Pain when standing on tiptoes, and sometimes pain when bending the knee. Swelling or bruising in the calf.

Complications if left unattended

Any strain left unattended can lead to a complete rupture. The calf muscle is used when standing and walking, so the pain could become disabling. A limp or change in gait due to this injury could lead to injury in other areas.

Immediate treatment

R.I.C.E.R. Anti-inflammatory medication. Then heat and massage to promote blood flow and healing.

Rehabilitation and prevention

As the pain subsides, a program of light stretching may help facilitate healing. When the pain has subsided, strengthening and stretching will help to prevent future injury. Proper warm-up before activities will help protect the muscle from tears. Strong flexible muscles resist strains better and recover more quickly.

Long-term prognosis

Muscle strains, when treated properly with rest and therapy, seldom have any lingering effects. In very rare cases where the muscle detaches completely, surgery may be required to re-attach the muscle.

093: ACHILLES TENDON STRAIN

Brief outline of injury

Achilles tendon strains can be very painful and take some time to heal. The Achilles tendon, which gets its name from the mythological Greek warrior *Achilles*, is located in the back of the lower leg over the heel. An injury to this tendon can be debilitating because of its involvement in walking and even balance during weight bearing. Explosive activities such as sprinting and jumping, and those activities that involve pushing against resistance such as football linemen and weight training, contribute greatly to this injury.

Anatomy and physiology

The Achilles tendon is the largest tendon in the human body, being approximately 15 cm long, and 2 cm thick. It originates from the musculo-tendinous junction of the calf muscles, and inserts into the posterior aspect of the calcaneus. The tendon is separated from the calcaneus by the *retrocalcaneal bursa*, and from the skin by the *subcutaneous calcaneal bursa*. It pulls the foot downward, extending it when the calf muscles contract. The strain can be graded on a scale from 1 to 3.
Grade 1 strain: A stretching or minor tear of the tendon (less than 25% of the tendon.)
Grade 2 strain: Involves more of the tendon fibres (usually 25% to 75%.)
Grade 3 strain: A complete rupture of the tendon.

Cause of injury

Abrupt, forceful contraction of the calf muscles; especially when the muscle and tendon are either cold or inflexible. Excessive force applied to the foot, forcing the foot into plantar flexion.

Signs and symptoms

Pain in the Achilles tendon, from mild discomfort in *grade 1 strains* to severe, debilitating pain in *grade 3 strains*. Swelling and tenderness may also be experienced. Pain when rising on the toes. Stiffness in the calf and heel area after resting.

Complications if left unattended

A minor tear may become a complete rupture if left unattended. Bursitis and tendinitis may develop from the inflamed tendon rubbing over the heel.

Immediate treatment

R.I.C.E.R. Anti-inflammatory medication. Then heat and massage to promote blood flow and healing. Immobilization and medical help for complete ruptures.

Rehabilitation and prevention

Rest is important and a gradual return to activity must be undertaken. Stretching and strengthening the calf muscles is important to rehabilitation and to prevent a recurrence. Warming-up the calf muscles properly before all activities, especially those involving forceful contractions such as sprinting, is essential to prevent strains.

Long-term prognosis

Due to the lower blood supply in tendons, they take longer to heal than the muscle, but with rest and rehabilitation, the Achilles tendon can return to normal function. Complete ruptures occasionally require surgical repair.

Rehabilitation exercises

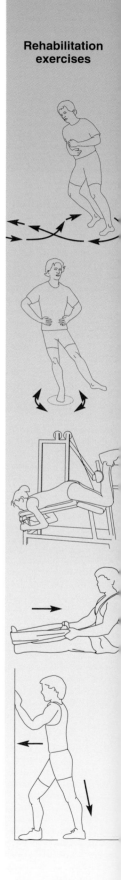

**Rehabilitation
exercises**

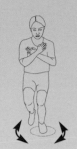

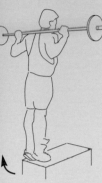

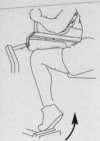

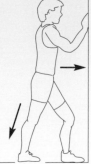

Brief outline of injury

Inflammation of the Achilles tendon can be very painful, especially since all of the body's weight is supported by this structure and the shoe often presses against this area. Repetitive stress to the tendon can lead to inflammation that causes additional irritation, causing more inflammation. Activities such as basketball, running, volleyball, and other running and jumping sports can lead to Achilles tendinitis.

Anatomy and physiology

The Achilles tendon is the largest tendon in the human body, being approximately 15 cm long, and 2 cm thick. It originates from the musculo-tendinous junction of the calf muscles and inserts into the posterior aspect of the calcaneus. The tendon is separated from the calcaneus by the retrocalcaneal bursa, and from the skin by the subcutaneous calcaneal bursa. The tendon crosses the back of the heel, which means it rides over the bone as the muscle contracts and stretches. Repetitive contraction of the muscles in the calf and improper footwear or excessive pronation of the feet can lead to inflammation in the tendon.

Cause of injury

Repetitive stress from running and jumping activities. Improper footwear or awkward landing pattern of the foot during running. Untreated injuries to the calf or Achilles tendon.

Signs and symptoms

Pain and tenderness in the tendon. Swelling may be present. Contraction of the calf muscle causes pain; running and jumping may be difficult.

Complications if left unattended

Inflammation in the tendon can lead to deterioration of the tendon and eventual rupture if left untreated. Inflammation may lead to tightening of the tendon and attached muscle, which could lead to tearing.

Immediate treatment

Rest, reducing or discontinuing the offending activity. Ice. Anti-inflammatory medication. Then heat and massage to promote blood flow and healing.

Rehabilitation and prevention

After a period of rest, usually lasting 5–10 days, gentle stretching and strengthening exercises can be initiated. Heat may be used on the tendon before activity to warm the tendon properly. Adequate warm-up, along with strengthening and stretching exercises for the calves, will help prevent tendinitis of the Achilles tendon.

Long-term prognosis

Tendinitis seldom has lingering effects if treated properly. Tendinitis may take from five days to several weeks to heal, but rarely needs surgery to repair it.

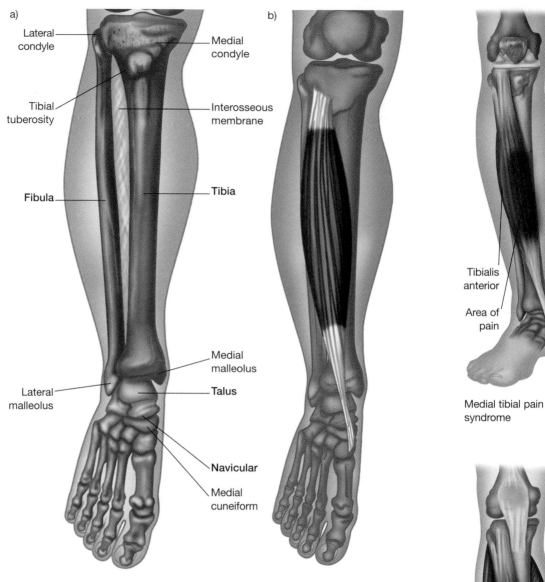

a)

Lateral condyle

Medial condyle

Tibial tuberosity

Interosseous membrane

Fibula

Tibia

Medial malleolus

Lateral malleolus

Talus

Navicular

Medial cuneiform

b)

Tibialis anterior

Area of pain

Medial tibial pain syndrome

Figure 15.3: The lower leg; a) anterior view, b) tibialis anterior muscle.

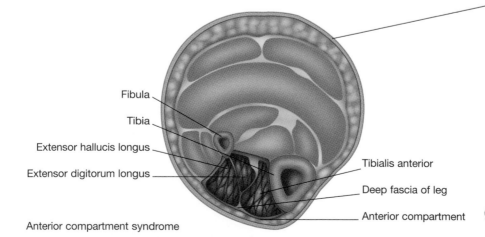

Fibula

Tibia

Extensor hallucis longus

Extensor digitorum longus

Tibialis anterior

Deep fascia of leg

Anterior compartment

Anterior compartment syndrome

Rehabilitation exercises

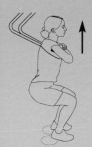

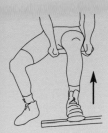

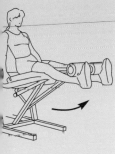

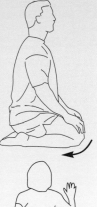

Brief outline of injury

Shin splints are a common complaint of runners and other athletes who have just taken up running. Shin splints are actually a term used to cover all pain in the anterior shin area. There are several possible causes. *Medial tibial pain syndrome*, the most common cause of shin pain, refers to pain felt over the shin bone from irritation of the tendons that cover the shin and their attachment to the bones. Changes in duration, frequency or intensity of running can lead to this condition.

Anatomy and physiology

The tibialis anterior muscle originates from the lateral condyle of the tibia, and inserts into the medial and plantar surfaces of the medial cuneiform bone. Tibialis anterior is responsible for dorsiflexing and inverting the foot and is used frequently during running to *toe up* with each step. When the muscle and tendon becomes inflamed and irritated through overuse or improper form, it will cause pain in the front of the shin. Repetitive pounding on the lower leg, such as with running, can also lead to pain in the shin.

Cause of injury

Repetitive stress on the tibialis anterior muscle leading to inflammation. Repetitive pounding force on the tibia, as with running and jumping.

Signs and symptoms

Dull, aching pain over the inside of the tibia. Pain is worse with activity. Tenderness over the inner side of the tibia with possible slight swelling.

Complications if left unattended

If left unattended, shin splints can cause extreme pain and cause cessation of running activities. The inflammation can lead to other injuries, including *compartment syndrome*.

Immediate treatment

R.I.C.E.R. Anti-inflammatory medication. Then heat and massage to promote blood flow and healing.

Rehabilitation and prevention

It is important to use low impact activities, such as swimming or cycling, to maintain conditioning levels while recovering. Stretching of the tibialis anterior muscle will help with recovery. To prevent this condition from developing, try alternating high impact activity days with lower impact days. It is also important to strengthen the muscles of the lower leg to help absorb the shock of impact activities.

Long-term prognosis

Medial tibial pain syndrome can be effectively treated with no long-term effects. Only in rare cases does the condition fail to respond to rest and rehabilitation, leading to chronic inflammation and pain. Surgery may be required in those rare cases.

096: STRESS FRACTURE

Brief outline of injury

Repetitive impact activities, such as running and jumping, can cause small cracks in the bone called *stress fractures*. These most often occur in the weight bearing bone, the tibia, of the lower leg. Athletes with lower bone density, due to dietary issues or genetic predisposition, are more susceptible, as are athletes who train on hard surfaces at increased distance and duration. Women are more susceptible to this injury than men due to bone density deficiency conditions such as irregular or absent menstrual cycles, eating disorders or osteoporosis.

Anatomy and physiology

The tibia *(shin bone)* is the larger and more medial of the bones in the lower leg. At the proximal end, the *medial* and *lateral condyles* articulate with the distal end of the femur to form the knee joint. The *tibial tuberosity* is a roughened area on the anterior surface of the tibia. The tibia is the weight bearing bone of the lower leg and therefore takes a large amount of the force of impact during running and jumping activities. This force is transferred up the length of the bone. Bones are constantly repairing and rebuilding, leading to the robbing of calcium from one area of the bone to build another, causing a weak area. When the impact is transferred up the shaft and encounters a weak area, due to either calcium deficiency or a prior stress fracture, the bone will crack slightly. Overtime, this leads to a more serious crack or fracture. Fatigued muscles also contribute to the possibility of stress fractures. The muscles are meant to take some of the shock away from the bones but a fatigued muscle is a poor shock absorber.

Cause of injury

Repetitive stress on the bone through impact activities such as running or jumping. Low bone density. Muscle fatigue leading to lower shock absorption by the muscles.

Signs and symptoms

Pain with weight bearing, worsens with activity and diminishes with rest. Pain is most severe at the early stage of activity, subsiding in the middle and returning at the end. Point tenderness and some swelling possible.

Complications if left unattended

If left unattended, a stress fracture can become a complete fracture and lead to complications such as bleeding and nerve compromise. The pain from an untreated stress fracture may lead to a complete cessation of activity and further injury to surrounding tissues.

Immediate treatment

R.I.C.E.R. Anti-inflammatory medication. If any instability is noted in the lower leg, or inability to bear weight, a sports medicine professional should be consulted.

Rehabilitation and prevention

During the recovery phase, it is important to maintain fitness levels by using low or non-impact activities such as swimming or biking. Strengthening the muscles of the lower leg will help add extra shock absorption. Warming-up properly and using cross training techniques to limit the impact of the bone will help prevent stress fractures.

Long-term prognosis

Stress fractures generally heal completely with rest. Returning to activity too soon may cause a recurrence. Very rarely surgical intervention may be needed to strengthen the bone at the fracture site.

Rehabilitation exercises

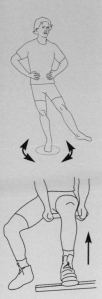

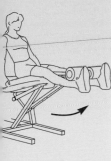

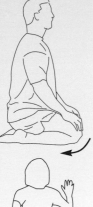

Brief outline of injury

Anterior compartment syndrome is more often a chronic rather than an acute injury. Runners and other athletes involved in activities that require a lot of repetitive flexion and extension of the foot are most susceptible. Swelling or enlargement of the muscle in the front of the lower leg, causes this condition. Pain, especially when *toeing up,* and decreased sensation and weakness in the foot may be experienced with this condition. Virtually any injury involving bleeding or oedema formation may lead to compartment syndrome.

Anatomy and physiology

Muscles are covered by *fascia*, a fairly inflexible fibrous sleeve that encases the muscle and bone. This creates a compartment for the muscle, with the bone forming one side, and the fascia covering the other sides. In the lower leg, the two bones, the *tibia* and the *fibula*, create a more rigid compartment. The *tibialis anterior* muscle runs over the tibia and fibula and is covered by the fascia. This leaves little room for expansion or swelling of the muscle. When there is increased intramuscular swelling, as a result of trauma or overuse, it creates pressure inside the compartment, which can impede blood flow and function of tissues within the compartment of the muscle.

Cause of injury

Acute: Trauma to, or tearing of, the tibialis anterior muscle causing bleeding and/or swelling. *Chronic*: Overuse of the muscle causing inflammation and swelling of the muscle and pressure in the compartment. Rapid growth of the muscle before the fascia can expand (as seen with anabolic steroid use).

Signs and symptoms

Pain and tightness in the shin (especially the lateral side). Worsens with exercise. Decreased sensation on top of the foot over the second toe. Weakness and tingling may be noticed in the foot.

Complications if left unattended

The pressure in the compartment may lead to permanent nerve and blood vessel damage if left unattended. The underlying cause of the condition will most likely continue to cause irritation and swelling if not treated.

Immediate treatment

Rest, ice and elevation (no compression). Anti-inflammatory medication. Sports massage may be used to stretch the fascia.

Rehabilitation and prevention

Stretching the muscles in the front of the shin will help to alleviate some of the pressure and elongate the muscle. Massage to stretch the fascia may also help to speed recovery. Gradual strengthening and a good flexibility program will help prevent this condition. Avoiding direct trauma to the shin area will prevent acute compartment syndrome.

Long-term prognosis

If treated before damage to the nerves and blood vessels becomes serious, the recovery rate is very good. Acute or severe chronic anterior compartment syndrome may require surgical intervention to relieve the pressure in the compartment.

Chapter

16

Sports Injuries of the
Ankle

Acute

098: Ankle Sprain

099: Ankle Fracture

Chronic

100: Posterior Tibial Tendinitis

101: Peroneal Tendon Subluxation

102: Peroneal Tendinitis

103: Osteochondritis Dissecans

104: Supination

105: Pronation

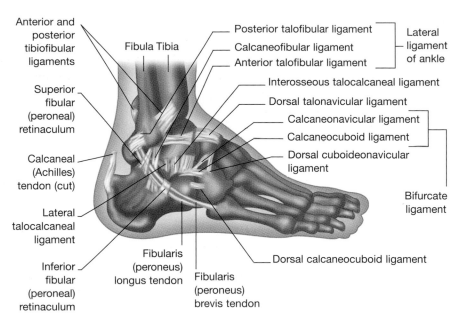

Anterior and posterior tibiofibular ligaments

Fibula Tibia

Posterior talofibular ligament

Calcaneofibular ligament

Anterior talofibular ligament

Lateral ligament of ankle

Superior fibular (peroneal) retinaculum

Interosseous talocalcaneal ligament

Dorsal talonavicular ligament

Calcaneonavicular ligament

Calcaneocuboid ligament

Dorsal cuboideonavicular ligament

Calcaneal (Achilles) tendon (cut)

Bifurcate ligament

Lateral talocalcaneal ligament

Inferior fibular (peroneal) retinaculum

Fibularis (peroneus) longus tendon

Fibularis (peroneus) brevis tendon

Dorsal calcaneocuboid ligament

Figure 16.1: The right ankle, lateral view.

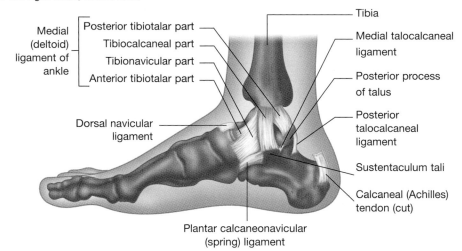

Medial (deltoid) ligament of ankle

Posterior tibiotalar part

Tibiocalcaneal part

Tibionavicular part

Anterior tibiotalar part

Tibia

Medial talocalcaneal ligament

Posterior process of talus

Posterior talocalcaneal ligament

Dorsal navicular ligament

Sustentaculum tali

Calcaneal (Achilles) tendon (cut)

Plantar calcaneonavicular (spring) ligament

Figure 16.2: The right ankle, medial view.

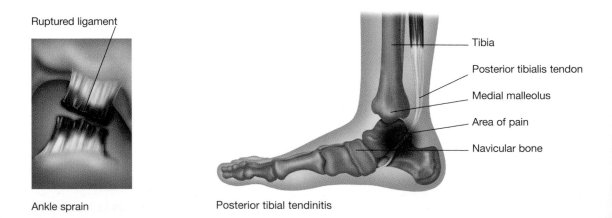

Ruptured ligament

Ankle sprain

Tibia

Posterior tibialis tendon

Medial malleolus

Area of pain

Navicular bone

Posterior tibial tendinitis

098: ANKLE SPRAIN

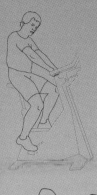

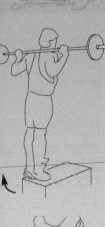

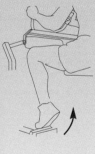

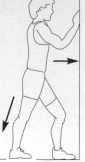

Brief outline of injury

Anyone involved in athletics is susceptible to an ankle sprain, an acute injury to any or all of the ligaments that support the ankle structure. Tearing or stretching of the ligaments can occur when the foot is rolled either medially or laterally, or twisted forcefully. High impact sports involving jumping, sprinting or running on changing or uneven surfaces often lead to ankle sprains. Basketball, football, cross country, and hockey are a few of the sports commonly associated with ankle sprains.

Anatomy and physiology

Lateral ankle sprains commonly occur when stress is applied to the ankle during plantar flexion and inversion, injuring the *anterior talofibular ligament*. The *medial malleolus* may act as a fulcrum to further invert the *calcaneofibular ligament* if the strain continues. The peroneal tendons may absorb some of this strain. *Medial ankle sprains* are less common, because of the strong *deltoid ligament* and bony structure of the ankle. The ligaments are stretched beyond their normal range and some tearing of the fibres may occur. Forceful twisting or rolling of the ankle, as with landing on the outside of the foot, can stretch the ligaments past their stretch point.

Cause of injury

Sudden twisting of the foot. Rolling or force to the foot, most commonly laterally.

Signs and symptoms

First-degree sprains: Result in little or no swelling, mild pain, and stiffness in the joint.
Second-degree sprains; Commonly exhibit more swelling and stiffness, moderate to severe pain, difficulty with weight bearing, and some instability in the joint.
Third-degree sprains: Result in severe swelling and pain, inability to bear weight, instability in the joint, and loss of function in the joint.

Complications if left unattended

Chronic pain and instability in the ankle joint may result if left unattended. Loss of strength and flexibility, and possible loss of function may also result. Re-injuring the joint is much more likely as well.

Immediate treatment

R.I.C.E.R. *Second- and third-degree sprains* may require immobilization and should seek medical attention immediately.

Rehabilitation and prevention

Strengthening the muscles of the lower leg is important to prevent future sprains. Balance activities will help to increase proprioception (the body's awareness of movement and position of the body), and strengthen the weakened ligaments. Flexibility exercises to reduce stiffness and improve mobility are needed also. Bracing during the initial return to activity may be needed but should not replace strengthening and flexibility development.

Long-term prognosis

With proper rehabilitation and strengthening, the athlete should not experience any limitations. A slight increase in the probability of injuring that ankle may occur. Athletes who continue to experience difficulty with the ankle may need additional medical interventions, including, in rare cases, possible surgery to *tighten* the ligaments.

Brief outline of injury

The ankle joint is one of the most commonly injured joints in the body. The majority of athletes have experienced at least a minor sprain of the ankle. Ankle fractures are less common, but nonetheless more common than other fractures. Due to the ankles involvement in all running and jumping activities, it is very susceptible to injury. Running or jumping on uneven or changing surfaces can lead to ankle fractures. High impact sports such as football and rugby, where the possibility of forceful twisting of the ankle may occur, also have a high incidence of ankle fractures.

Anatomy and physiology

The ankle joint, is a hinge joint, and comprises the *tibia, fibula* and *talus* bones. The ankle joint articulates between the *distal tibia*, the *medial malleolus* of the tibia, the *lateral malleolus* of the fibula and the talus. These bones are held together by a series of ligaments. In an ankle fracture, any or all of the bones and ligaments may become involved. Ankle fractures most commonly involve the ends of the tibia or fibula, or both, with some ligament stretching and tearing present as well.

Cause of injury

Forceful twisting or rolling of the ankle can cause the end of the bones to fracture. Forceful impact to the medial or lateral side of the ankle while the foot is planted.

Signs and symptoms

Pain to touch. Swelling and discolouration. Inability to bear weight. Deformity may be present in the ankle joint.

Complications if left unattended

An ankle fracture that is left unattended can result in incorrect or incomplete healing of the bones. Continued walking or running on the injured ankle could result in further damage to the ligaments, blood vessels, and nerves that pass through the joint.

Immediate treatment

Stop the activity. Immobilize the joint and apply ice. Seek medical attention.

Rehabilitation and prevention

While the ankle is immobilized, it is important to keep conditioning levels up by using upper body exercises and weight training. When cleared for activity with the ankle, strengthening and stretching of the muscles of the lower leg is essential for a speedy recovery. An ankle brace may be needed for support during the initial return to activity. Stronger calf and anterior muscles help support the ankle and prevent or lessen the incidence of injuries. Avoid running and jumping on uneven surfaces as much as possible.

Long-term prognosis

Although people who have fractured their ankle tend to have a slightly higher rate of re-injury, proper strengthening and rehabilitation usually lead to a full recovery. Compound fractures or those in misalignment may require surgical pinning to hold the bone in place while it heals.

Rehabilitation exercises

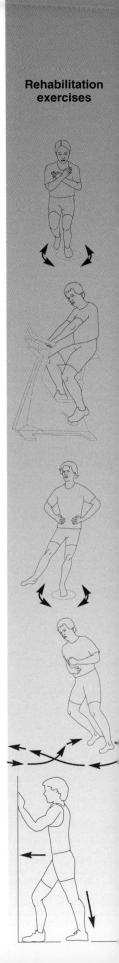

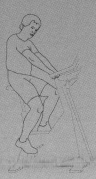

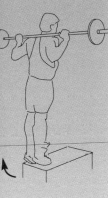

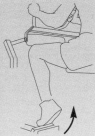

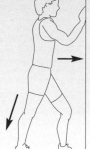

Brief outline of injury

Pain along the medial (inner) side of the lower leg, ankle, and foot may be the result of posterior tibial tendinitis. The posterior tibial tendon helps hold the longitudinal arch of the foot, which means there is a level of tension and friction in the tendon. If the arch falls, the stress on the tendon will increase. This can occur with poor running mechanics, improper footwear, or untreated injuries.

Anatomy and physiology

The posterior tibial tendon runs from the calf muscle behind the *medial malleolus* (the bony prominence) of the ankle, to the *navicular bone* in the arch of the foot. This tendon supports the arch and aids in inversion of the foot. If the navicular moves out of place, it causes stress and irritation to the tendon. This irritation over time becomes *tendinitis*, inflammation of the tendon.

Cause of injury

Improper running mechanics. Improper footwear. Prior injury to the medial side of the ankle.

Signs and symptoms

Pain and tenderness over the inner side of the shin, ankle, and foot. Pain when walking or running. Some swelling may be noted over the tendon.

Complications if left unattended

If left unattended, this condition can lead to a fallen arch or a complete rupture of the tendon. The pain may cause a change in footfall during running leading to injuries in other structures of the foot and ankle.

Immediate treatment

R.I.C.E.R. Anti-inflammatory medication.

Rehabilitation and prevention

After pain subsides, it is important to stretch and strengthen the calf muscles to support the tendon and speed recovery. Arch supports may be required until the tendon heals and the muscles are strengthened. Gradual reintroduction into activity is important and proper warm-ups will help prevent a recurrence of the injury. Proper footwear and corrections of any mechanical inefficiency will also help prevent this injury.

Long-term prognosis

Proper treatment should lead to a complete recovery. The longer the condition exists before treatment the longer recovery will take. In some cases orthotics may be required to prevent a recurrence.

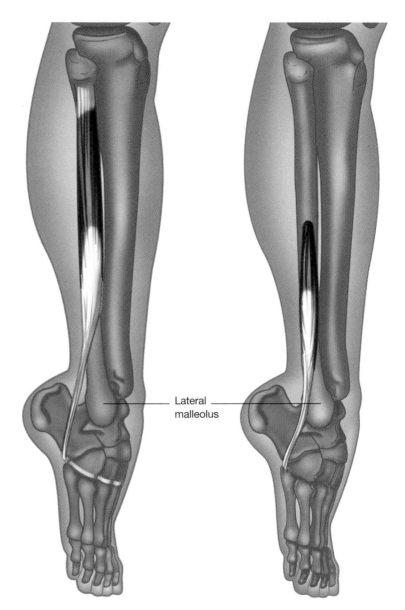

Lateral malleolus

Figure 16.3: Peroneus longus and peroneus brevis, right leg, lateral view.

Bone

Inflamed tendon

Muscle

Area of pain

Fibularis (peroneus) longus tendon

Peroneal tendon subluxation

Peroneal tendinitis

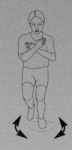

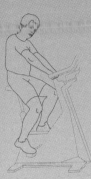

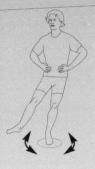

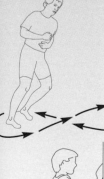

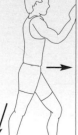

Brief outline of injury

Peroneal tendon subluxation (dislocation) is most commonly a chronic condition that develops after a sprain or fracture. The tendon moves out of the groove in which it is supposed to sit due to damage to the structures designed to hold it in place. Pain on the lateral side (outside) of the ankle and a popping sensation may be signs of this condition. Running and jumping can cause repetitive stress to the tendon, especially when it is dislocating repetitively.

Anatomy and physiology

The tendons of *peroneus longus* and *peroneus brevis* run from the peroneal muscles to the foot. They pass around the *lateral malleolus* through a groove in the bone. They are held in this groove sheath that is reinforced by a band of ligament. When this ligament or sheath is damaged, it reduces the stability of the tendons, allowing movement out of the groove. Some people are predisposed to this injury due to a shallow, or non-existent groove where the tendons lie. Peroneal tendon subluxation may occur also if the tip of the lateral malleolus is fractured with forced dorsiflexion, or a direct blow.

Cause of injury

Tearing or stretching of the ligaments that support the tendons, usually due to an ankle sprain or fracture. Repetitive stress to the tendons, causing inflammation and swelling, allowing the tendons to slide out of the groove.

Signs and symptoms

Pain and tenderness along the tendons. Popping or snapping sensation on the lateral side of the ankle. Swelling may be noted along the bottom of the fibula.

Complications if left unattended

The peroneal tendons become irritated when they dislocate, which causes inflammation. This inflammation can lead to tearing or complete rupture of the tendons if left untreated.

Immediate treatment

R.I.C.E.R. Anti-inflammatory medication. Possible immobilization, especially with acute dislocation.

Rehabilitation and prevention

Strengthening of the muscles in the lower leg after pain subsides and normal function returns will help support the tendons. Treating ankle sprains properly will help prevent subluxation. Strong calf and shin muscles will help support the whole foot and ankle structure, preventing this condition as well.

Long-term prognosis

When treated promptly, subluxation of the peroneal tendons usually responds well to non-surgical techniques. In some cases, surgery may be required to repair the sheath and ligaments that cover the tendon to restore stability.

SPORTS INJURIES OF THE ANKLE

Brief outline of injury

The peroneal tendon is involved in stabilizing the foot and providing support to the ankle to prevent lateral rolling of the joint. When the foot pronates it causes the tendon to stretch leading to pain and inflammation. The tendon has to work harder to stabilize the foot during pronation. Runners who have excessive pronation often develop this condition.

Anatomy and physiology

The tendons of *peroneus longus* and *peroneus brevis* run from the peroneal muscles to the foot. They pass around the *lateral malleolus* (the bony prominence on the outside of the ankle) and attach just behind the big toe. These tendons, along with the peroneal muscles, help to stabilize the foot and assist the calf muscles to extend the foot. When the foot pronates causing the tendons to stretch, it puts extra stress on the tendons, leading to pain and inflammation. Running and jumping cause repetitive flexing of the peroneal muscles and can lead to inflammation of the tendons, especially with excessive pronation.

Cause of injury

Over-pronation of the foot during running or jumping. Prior ankle injury leading to an incorrect path of travel for the tendons.

Signs and symptoms

Pain and tenderness along the tendons. Pain is most severe at the beginning of the activity and diminishes as the activity continues. Gradual increase in pain overtime.

Complications if left unattended

Unattended tendinitis can lead to a complete rupture of the tendons. Peroneal tendinitis can lead to subluxations. The chronic inflammation can also lead to damage to the ligaments surrounding the tendons.

Immediate treatment

Rest, especially from running or jumping activities. Ice. Anti-inflammatory medication.

Rehabilitation and prevention

Stretching of the calf muscles and a gradual reintroduction into activity is important for rehabilitation. During the recovery period it is important to identify and correct any foot or gait problems that may be contributing to the problem. Prevention of this condition requires strong, flexible muscles of the lower leg to support the foot and ankle.

Long-term prognosis

With proper treatment, peroneal tendinitis will usually heal completely with no lingering effects. In rare cases, the tendinitis may not respond to traditional treatment and may require surgical intervention to relieve the pressure causing the inflammation. Arch supporting orthotics may be required in some cases as well.

Rehabilitation exercises

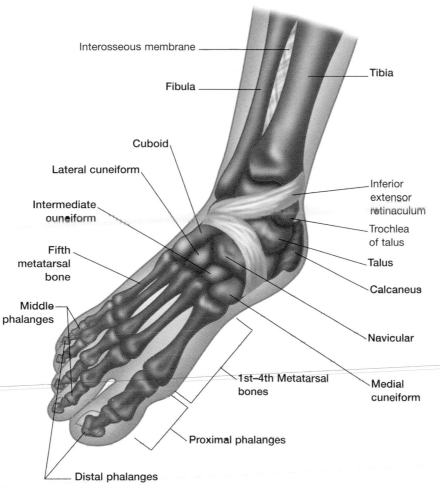

Figure 16.4: The bones of the right foot, anteromedial view.

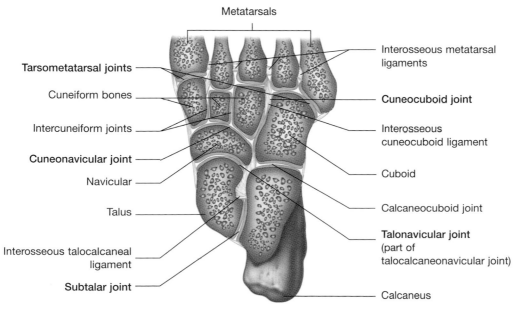

Figure 16.5: The intertarsal joints (horizontal section of the right foot).

103: OSTEOCHONDRITIS DISSECANS

Brief outline of injury

Osteochondritis dissecans (loose bodies in the joint) occurs when a fragment of bone adjacent to the articular surface of a joint is deprived of its blood supply, leading to avascular necrosis. This causes the cartilage to become brittle and a piece, or pieces, may break off. If the cartilage gets into the joint, it can cause pain and inflammation. The space in the ankle joint is very small and when a bone or cartilage fragment from the talus bone gets lodged in the joint, it can cause pain, swelling, and loss of movement in the ankle. These symptoms may come and go as the free-floating fragment floats in and out of the joint. Prior ankle injuries make a person susceptible to this condition, as does any blockage of blood flow to the feet.

Anatomy and physiology

The tarsals are the seven bones of the ankle. The two largest tarsals carry the body weight: the *calcaneus*, or the heel bone, and the *talus*, which lies between the *tibia* and the calcaneus. The *tibia* and *fibula* rest on top of the talus. The articular surface of the talus is covered with cartilage to cushion and protect it. There is very little blood flow to this area so repairing damage is difficult for the body. This can result in the tissue becoming brittle and breaking off. A fracture can occur on the surface of the talus, or the cartilage may become bruised from any twisting injury causing the talus to come in hard contact with the tibia or fibula.

Cause of injury

Loss of blood flow to the articular surface of the talus along with injury to the bone. Repetitive wear on the cartilage and bone surface of the talus. Previous ankle injury.

Signs and symptoms

Pain and discomfort in the joint. If the fragment becomes detached and lodged in the joint, swelling and loss of movement may occur. A catching sensation in the ankle may be felt.

Complications if left unattended

The loose bodies in the joint can cause scarring and additional damage if left unattended. As the joint moves and the loose body grinds against the other cartilage and bone surfaces, it will wear at these surfaces making them rough and eventually lead to arthritis.

Immediate treatment

Rest and possible immobilization of the joint. Referral to a sports medicine professional. Anti-inflammatory medication.

Rehabilitation and prevention

Rehabilitating the ankle after this type of injury includes strengthening the muscles of the lower leg to offer additional support to the joint. Stretching and range of motion activities may be required if the ankle was immobilized for treatment. Gradual return to activity will help to prevent it from recurring immediately. Treating all ankle injuries properly, no matter how minor, will help prevent the blood flow loss and protect the talus.

Long-term prognosis

Many times the loose body does not detach from the bone, allowing the body to heal itself. If it does become detached, it may require surgical removal. If allowed to wear at the joint, it could lead to osteoarthritis, especially in the older athlete.

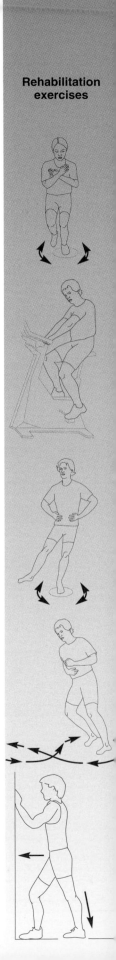

Rehabilitation exercises

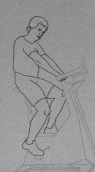

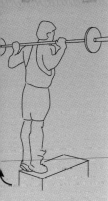

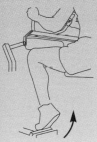

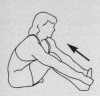

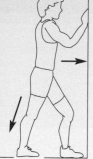

Brief outline of injury

Supination is the *outward* rolling of the foot at the ankle. This is a normal movement during the push-off phase of running, walking, or jumping. Excessive supination can cause damage to the ligaments, tendons, and muscles of the lower leg. Acute over-supination may cause stretching or tearing of the ligaments of the foot and ankle. Excessive supination can lead to a weakening of the ankle structure and decreased stability.

Anatomy and physiology

Supination involves the bones of the ankle joint, but more specifically, the *subtalar joint*. The distal (lower) ends of the tibia and fibula rest on the talus of the foot and allow for movement of the foot. This is traditionally referred to as a *hinge joint* because its main function is to allow flexion and extension of the foot. It does, however, allow limited pronation and supination as well, which is normal during running, walking, and jumping. These movements aid balance and improve shock absorption.

Cause of injury

Weak or loose tendons and ligaments in the ankle. Weak or fatigued muscles of the lower leg. Forceful outward rolling of the ankle. Improper or worn footwear. Uneven or sloped running (or landing) surface.

Signs and symptoms

Pain in the arch, heel, and/or knees and hips. Instability in the ankle. Pain over the outside of the ankle. Pain may be immediate with acute over-supination (such as an ankle sprain).

Complications if left unattended

May lead to chronic weakness and instability in the ankle. The pain and improper gait may lead to compensation and injury to other structures and tissues. The ligaments may lose their elasticity from excessive stretching, and tearing may occur.

Immediate treatment

Rest, ice, and anti-inflammatory medications to help alleviate the pain. Acute over-supination may require medical attention and immobilization. Chronic supination will require correction of the underlying problems, whilst allowing adequate rest for the tissues to recover.

Rehabilitation and prevention

Proper warm-up is essential. Strengthening and stretching of the muscles of the lower leg may help support the ankle, keep it moving in the correct plane, and reduce excessive supination. Orthotics and gait analysis may be required. Gradual return to a full workload is recommended and retraining of the athlete to improve, or correct running form is important. Ensure proper footwear and a smooth flat running (or landing) surface.

Long-term prognosis

Will respond well if treated early with a good rehabilitation plan. The length of time the condition is allowed to persist will also affect the recovery time. In rare cases, surgery may be required to tighten the tendons or correct skeletal factors.

Brief outline of injury

Pronation is the *inward* rotation of the foot during walking or running. While some pronation is natural and part of the normal gait, excessive pronation can lead to some chronic injuries, and acute over-pronation can lead to strains or sprains.

Anatomy and physiology

The ankle is a *hinge joint* and is formed of the seven tarsal bones. The two largest tarsals carry the body weight: the *calcaneus*, or the heel bone, and the *talus*, which lies between the tibia and the calcaneus. The *tibia* and *fibula* rest on top of the talus. Pronation occurs at the subtalar joint. The strong ligaments of the ankle help provide support and prevent excessive pronation. The muscles of the calf and the anterior muscles of the lower leg also offer support. When these ligaments are loose or the muscles fatigue, the support is lost, which results in more pronation. This causes the arch of the foot to flatten out, which in turn further stretches the ligaments. Also, during weight bearing at midstance, there is a tendency for calcaneal eversion and foot abduction, as the foot moves into dorsiflexion.

Cause of injury

Loose or torn tendons from previous ankle injuries. Weak or fatigued muscles of the lower leg. Improper or worn footwear. Uneven running (or landing) surfaces.

Signs and symptoms

Pain in the arch, heel, and/or knees and hips. Pain during the landing phase of running or jumping. Visible inward rolling of the foot and ankle. Instability in the ankle. Pain may be immediate for acute over-pronation, such as an ankle sprain, or gradual for chronic pronation disorders.

Complications if left unattended

Pronation has been attributed to shin splints, plantar fasciitis, chondromalacia patellae, tendinitis, and even stress fractures. The longer pronation continues, the more the ligaments of the foot and ankle will be stretched, leading to ankle instability. The arches may flatten out and lead to other problems of the foot. Chronic pronation of the foot beyond normal ranges can lead to overuse and chronic injuries.

Immediate treatment

Rest, ice and anti-inflammatory medications may help alleviate the pain. For acute injuries, immobilization and reduction of weight bearing activities may be required. For chronic injuries, seek the help of a qualified sports medicine specialist to help identify and correct the problem.

Rehabilitation and prevention

Correct the underlying problem, e.g. if due to the running surface, change the surface to one that is flat or smooth. If due to footwear, try some new or different shoes. If necessary, use orthotics and gait training. Warm-up properly. Stretching and strengthening will offer support and keep the muscles of the lower leg strong and flexible. Completely rehabilitate any ankle injury before returning to sport to prevent any re-occurrence.

Long-term prognosis

Will usually respond well to treatment, although the longer pronation goes untreated and allowed to cause damage to the ligaments, the longer the recovery time. In very rare cases, surgical intervention may be required to correct any underlying orthopedic issues.

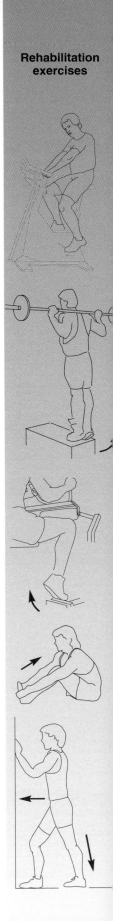

Chapter
17

Sports Injuries of the Foot

Acute

106: Fracture of the Foot

Chronic

107: Retrocalcaneal Bursitis

108: Stress Fracture

109: Extensor and Flexor Tendinitis

110: Morton's Neuroma

111: Sesamoiditis

112: Bunions

113: Hammer Toe

114: Turf Toe

115: Claw Foot (Pes Cavus)

116: Plantar Fasciitis

117: Heel Spur

118: Black Nail (Subungual Haematoma)

119: Ingrown Toenail

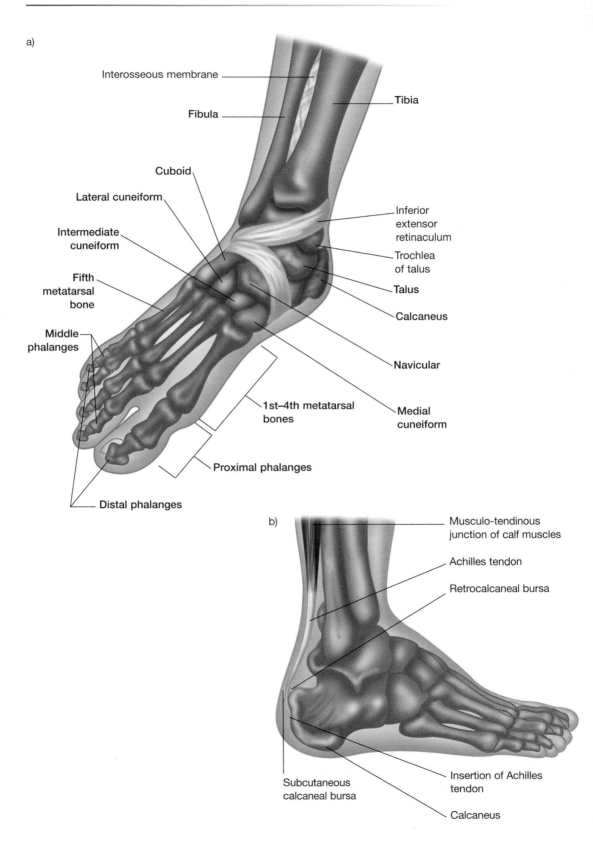

Figure 17.1: a) The bones of the right foot, anteromedial view, b) Achilles tendon.

106: FRACTURE OF THE FOOT

Rehabilitation exercises

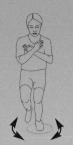

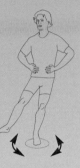

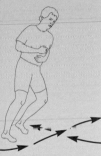

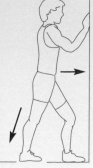

Brief outline of injury

A foot fracture may involve any of the twenty-six bones of the foot but most commonly occurs in the metatarsals. Contact sports and those that could result in high impact landing or collisions can lead to foot fractures. Those athletes with lower bone density due to poor nutrition, osteoporosis, (or inadequate or absent menstrual cycles in females) are more susceptible to fractures.

Anatomy and physiology

The foot consists of twenty-six small bones. The seven tarsals form the ankle. The two largest tarsals carry the body weight: the *calcaneus*, or the heel bone, and the *talus*, which lies between the tibia and the calcaneus. The *tibia* and *fibula* rest on top of the talus. The five *metatarsals* are long, narrow bones that form the instep or sole of the foot and the fourteen *phalanges* consist of short, narrow bones that form the toes, with two joints in the big toe and three in the others. These bones, due to their location and shape, are more susceptible to fracture. When a force is applied to the shaft of the metatarsals, they may fracture.

Cause of injury

Trauma to the bones of the foot, e.g. fall, blow, collision, or violent twisting.

Signs and symptoms

Pain, which can be severe. Swelling and discolouration, and possible deformity at the fracture site. Pain when weight bearing, and possible inability to walk. Numbness of the foot or toes.

Complications if left unattended

A fracture that is left untreated can lead to damage to the blood vessels and nerves in and around the fracture site. The bones may heal incorrectly or not heal at all. Weakness and instability in the foot may result as well.

Immediate treatment

Immediate removal from activity. Ice, elevation, and possible immobilization. Consult with a sports medicine professional or make an emergency room visit.

Rehabilitation and prevention

After pain subsides and normal function returns, stretching of the muscles that were not used during recovery is important. Strengthening of the muscles that likely have atrophied due to lack of use during immobilization is also a must. Strong muscles to support the foot are essential to prevent foot fractures. Avoiding direct trauma to the foot is the best tool for prevention. Proper footwear to offer support and protection will also help prevent this injury.

Long-term prognosis

If allowed to heal completely, a fracture will usually heal to become stronger than before the injury. In fractures that are *compound* or *misaligned*, surgical pinning may be required to stabilize the bone until it heals. If the ligaments are stretched or torn, the chance of re-injury increases.

Rehabilitation exercises

Brief outline of injury

The retrocalcaneal bursa helps to lubricate and cushion the tendon as it runs over the heel. This bursa takes a lot of stress during repetitive flexing and extending of the foot, such as during running, walking, or jumping. Worn or incorrectly sized footwear or excessive pronation of the foot can also lead to problems with this bursa, as well as the Achilles tendon. Shoes that fit too tightly, especially in the back, may put additional stress on the tendon and bursa.

Anatomy and physiology

The retrocalcaneal bursa lies between the anterior *Achilles tendon* insertion and the *calcaneus* (heel bone). The repetitive friction of the tendon running over this bursa during active plantar flexion during push-off compresses the bursa between the tendon and bone, and can cause inflammation.

Cause of injury

Repetitive stress to the bursa by the friction of the Achilles tendon during walking, running, or jumping. Increasing duration or distance too quickly. Improper footwear or walking/running gait. Injury to the Achilles tendon.

Signs and symptoms

Pain, especially with walking, running, or jumping. Tenderness over the heel area. Redness and slight swelling may be noted over the heel.

Complications if left unattended

The bursa can rupture completely if the injury is left unattended. This complete rupture could lead to other problems with the Achilles tendon due to increased friction. The pain may make it difficult to get up on the toes during walking, running, or jumping.

Immediate treatment

Rest from activities that cause pain. Ice. Anti-inflammatory medication.

Rehabilitation and prevention

Strengthening the muscles of the calf and stretching the muscles of the lower leg will help facilitate healing. Using activities that do not irritate the area to maintain fitness levels is essential. Keeping the muscles strong and flexible and allowing adequate warm-up before all activities will help prevent bursitis.

Long-term prognosis

Proper treatment and rest should lead to a complete recovery. In rare cases the fluid that builds up due to the inflammation may need to be drained to facilitate healing. Surgery is only necessary in extreme cases that do not respond to rest and rehabilitation.

Rehabilitation exercises

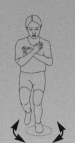

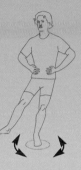

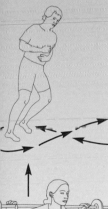

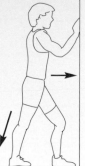

Brief outline of injury

Stress fractures in the foot are usually a result of repetitive impact to the bones of the feet. Running or jumping on hard surfaces, changing the duration or distance of workouts too quickly, or fatigued muscles that can no longer absorb shock can lead to small cracks in the bone. The small cracks accumulate and become a *stress fracture*.

Anatomy and physiology

A stress fracture can occur in any of the bones of the foot but are generally seen in the *metatarsals*. The heel bone, or *calcaneus*, can also become fractured with improper footwear or as the result of an old injury that has gone untreated. The bones subjected to repetitive trauma develop minor cracks and then these cracks build on each other leading to a stress fracture. A weak point in the bone from a previous injury or due to bone rebuilding can lead to stress fractures under normal stress conditions.

Cause of injury

Repetitive trauma to the bones of the foot. Weakened area of bone due to previous injury or other condition. Muscle fatigue, making the muscles ineffective shock absorbers.

Signs and symptoms

Pain at the site of the fracture. Pain with weight bearing, with inability to walk in severe cases. Swelling may be noted over the fracture site. Some loss of foot function may be noted.

Complications if left unattended

More serious stress fracture including a complete break in the bone may occur if left unattended. Swelling and inflammation may cause blood flow and nerve problems in the foot. Pain may increase to the point of disability and inability to walk.

Immediate treatment

R.I.C.E.R. Anti-inflammatory medication.

Rehabilitation and prevention

Strengthening of the muscles that support the foot will help to lessen the impact on the foot, with stronger muscles absorbing more shock. A gradual start to activity after the injury has healed is important to prevent recurrence. Proper footwear, correct warm-up techniques, avoiding hard running surfaces and a diet with calcium-rich foods will help prevent stress fractures in the foot.

Long-term prognosis

Stress fractures will usually heal completely and have no lingering effects if rest and rehabilitation are used. The fracture site should heal to become stronger than it was originally. Only in severe cases where the bone fractures completely and does not respond to rest and immobilization, will surgery be required.

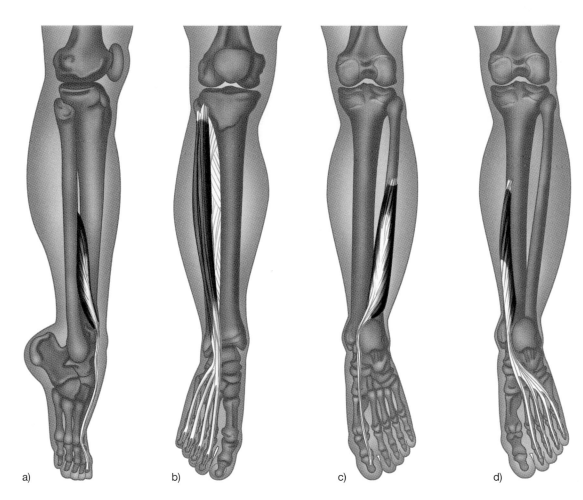

a) b) c) d)

Figure 17.2: The extensor and flexor muscles of the foot.

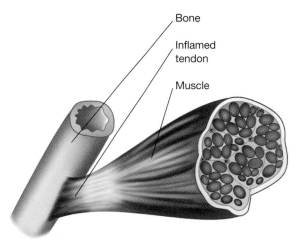

Bone

Inflamed
tendon

Muscle

Flexor and extensor tendinitis

Rehabilitation exercises

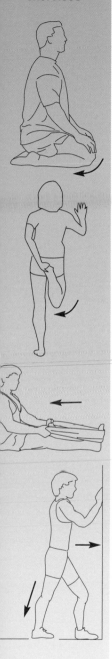

Brief outline of injury

The tendons attached to the muscles that are responsible for flexing and extending the toes and foot can become inflamed and irritated just like any other tendon. Overuse, tightness in opposing muscles, or foot deformities can cause this condition. Extensor tendinitis is more common than flexor, but flexor tendinitis tends to be more painful and debilitating. Dancers are most commonly associated with injury to this tendon group.

Anatomy and physiology

The *extensor hallucis longus* (a) and *extensor digitorum longus* (b) are the main extensor muscles of the toes. The tendons of these muscles run over the front of the ankle, over the foot and attach to the toes. These muscles dorsiflex the foot and work in opposition to the flexor muscles. When the calf muscles are tight, or the muscles are worked beyond their exertion level, inflammation of the tendon may occur.

The flexor group of muscles, the *flexor hallucis longus* (c) and the *flexor digitorum longus* (d), have tendons that run down the inside of the ankle and under the foot, attaching to the toes. These muscles plantar flex the foot and toes.

Cause of injury

Extensor tendinitis: Tight calf muscles, over-exertion of the extensor muscles, or fallen arches.
Flexor tendinitis: Repetitive stress to the tendon from excessive dorsiflexion of the toes.

Signs and symptoms

Extensor tendinitis: Pain on the top of the foot, pain when dorsiflexing the toes, some strength loss may be experienced.
Flexor tendinitis: Pain along the tendon, in the arch of the foot, and along the inside back of the ankle.

Complications if left unattended

Tendinitis when left unattended can cause strains to the attached muscle and could lead to a complete rupture of the tendon. The pain may become severe enough to limit all activity.

Immediate treatment

Rest from activities that cause pain. Ice the tendon. Anti-inflammatory medication.

Rehabilitation and prevention

While resting the foot, it is important to identify the conditions that caused the problem. Stretching the calf muscles and the tibialis anterior muscle will help relieve the pressure on the tendons. Warming-up and gradually increasing workloads will help prevent tendinitis. Orthotics may be required when returning to activity to correct any arch problems.

Long-term prognosis

Most people recover completely from tendinitis with simple rest and correction of the cause(s). In some rare cases, surgery may be required to reduce the pressure on the tendons and relieve the inflammation.

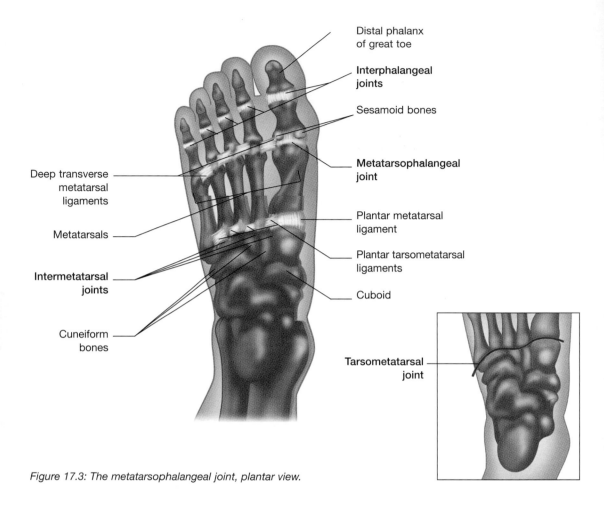

Figure 17.3: The metatarsophalangeal joint, plantar view.

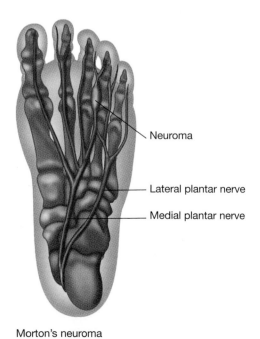

Morton's neuroma

Brief outline of injury

A neuroma is a tumour, growing from a nerve, or made up largely of nerve cells and nerve fibres. *Morton's neuroma* involves the plantar nerve, and is characterized by pain on the plantar side of the foot. When pressure is applied to the forefoot area, the bones may pinch the nerve causing pain, burning, or even loss of sensation to the affected area. Running (especially sprinting), walking, and jumping all place repetitive stress on this area and have the potential to cause Morton's neuroma. Foot deformities, underlying foot abnormalities, or tight-fitting shoes that compress the foot, can also lead to this condition.

Anatomy and physiology

The *plantar nerve* supplies the third and fourth toes, and runs between the *metatarsal heads*. When the bones are subjected to pressure due to tight-fitting shoes or a pronated foot, the plantar nerves become compressed between the metatarsal heads, which causes inflammation and swelling.

Cause of injury

Repetitive stress or trauma to the ball of the foot, such as with running, walking, or jumping. Pronation. Wearing footwear that compresses the foot. Injuries to the metatarsals of the third and fourth toe.

Signs and symptoms

Pain and/or burning sensation in the affected area. Possible loss of sensation in the third and fourth toes. Possible numbness, tingling, or cramping in the forefoot. While weight bearing in shoes, agonizing pain on the lateral side of the foot may be present, which is relieved when going barefoot.

Complications if left unattended

If left unattended, a neuroma may lead to permanent nerve damage. Permanent loss of sensation to the toes may also result. Pain will increase without treatment, eventually leading to disability.

Immediate treatment

Rest from, or modification of activity. Anti-inflammatory medication. Ice.

Rehabilitation and prevention

A gradual return to activity and avoiding repetitive trauma to the forefoot will help speed recovery. Padding may be needed when activity is resumed. The most important step in prevention of this condition is to use footwear that allows for plenty of room for the foot. Narrow toed shoes and high heels should be avoided.

Long-term prognosis

When treated properly, a neuroma should recover completely without any long-term effects. The longer the injury goes untreated, the higher the possibility for lingering effects. Surgery may be required if the regular treatment does not lead to recovery.

Brief outline of injury

The tendons surrounding the sesamoid bones can become irritated and inflamed, causing a condition similar to *tendinitis*. Runners, dancers, and catchers in baseball are all susceptible to this injury. Increasing activity too quickly causes additional trauma to the small sesamoid bones.

Anatomy and physiology

A sesamoid is a small nodular bone that is not attached to another bone, but instead is embedded in a tendon or joint. The knee cap is the largest sesamoid bone in the body but there are also two small ones in the forefoot. The *sesamoid bones* in the foot are located along the plantar surface of the first metatarsal head, with one on the lateral aspect, and the other more medial. The sesamoid bones are spherical and embedded in the tendon of the flexor hallucis brevis. They provide a smooth surface for the tendon to travel over and help the tendon to transmit the force generated by the muscles. The sesamoid bones in the foot also help elevate the bones of the big toe and assist in weight bearing.

Cause of injury

Increased activity without proper conditioning. Little natural padding in the forefoot, leaving the sesamoid bones unprotected. High arches leading to running on the balls of the feet.

Signs and symptoms

Gradual onset of pain. Pain over the bone and surrounding tendon. Pain increases with activity.

Complications if left unattended

If left unattended, this condition can worsen to the point that the pain becomes debilitating. The inflammation in the tendon can cause irritation to surrounding tissue. As with tendinitis, a complete rupture may occur if the condition is allowed to go untreated.

Immediate treatment

Rest. Ice. Anti-inflammatory medication.

Rehabilitation and prevention

Finding activities that do not stress or irritate the injured area will help to keep fitness levels up. Strengthening the muscles of the lower leg will help support the foot. Wearing padding inside the shoes may be necessary when returning to activity. Gradually increasing distance or duration will help prevent this condition, as will warming-up properly before beginning exercise. Orthotics or implants to correct arch problems may also help prevent sesamoiditis.

Long-term prognosis

Sesamoiditis responds well to rest and anti-inflammatory treatments. Complete recovery can be expected, with no lingering effects. In rare cases where the condition does not respond to preliminary treatments, surgical intervention may be required.

Rehabilitation exercises

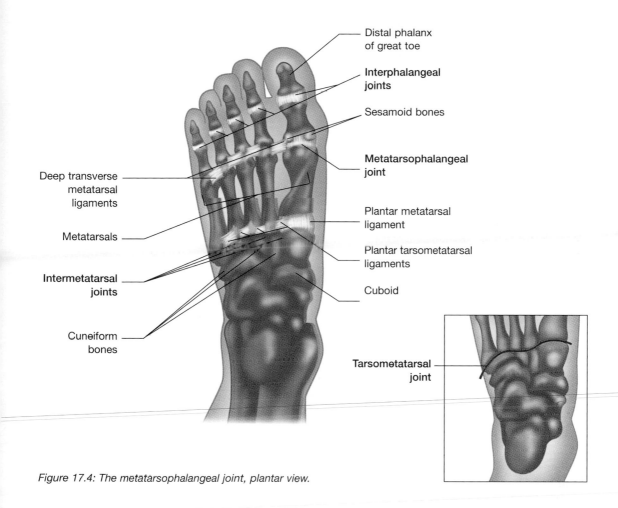

Distal phalanx
of great toe

**Interphalangeal
joints**

Sesamoid bones

**Metatarsophalangeal
joint**

Plantar metatarsal
ligament

Plantar tarsometatarsal
ligaments

Cuboid

Tarsometatarsal
joint

Deep transverse
metatarsal
ligaments

Metatarsals

**Intermetatarsal
joints**

Cuneiform
bones

Figure 17.4: The metatarsophalangeal joint, plantar view.

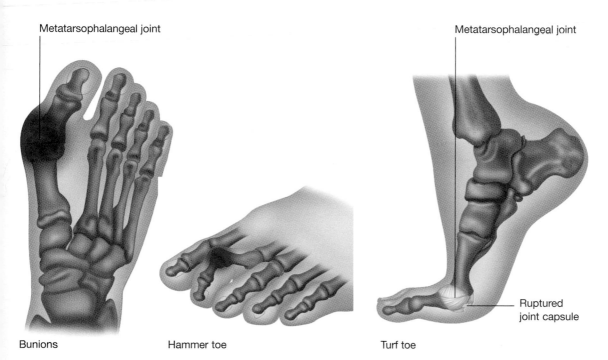

Metatarsophalangeal joint

Metatarsophalangeal joint

Ruptured
joint capsule

Bunions

Hammer toe

Turf toe

Brief outline of injury

Tight-fitting or ill-fitting shoes can lead to swelling and enlarging of the joint at the base of the big toe, known as a *bunion*. Injury to the big toe or abnormal stress on the outside of the toe can also lead to bunions. Women are much more likely to get bunions than men, due to the tendency of females to wear tighter fitting shoes. A bunion-like condition may develop on the lateral (small toe) aspect of the foot called a *bunionette*.

Anatomy and physiology

Bunions are typically found on the medial aspect of the *metatarsophalangeal joint*, which connects the toe and foot. When tight-fitting shoes, an injury, or other condition causes pressure on the toe (forcing it inward), the joint becomes inflamed and enlarged. There is inflammation of the bursa overlying the medial aspect of the first metatarsal head. This causes the toe to move laterally toward the second toe, sometimes even sliding under it, forming the *hallux valgus* deformity. A painful bump develops on the outside of the toe joint, which leads to additional pain and inflammation.

Cause of injury

Tight-fitting shoes. Untreated injury to the big toe. Unusual pressure to the outside of the first toe. Pronation of the foot.

Signs and symptoms

Bump at the base of the big toe. The first toe may move laterally toward the second toe. Redness and tenderness in the affected area. Pain with walking.

Complications if left unattended

Bunions left unattended may lead to further complications such as bursitis, difficulty walking, arthritis, and chronic pain. The first toe may angle toward the second toe causing the second toe to move out of alignment.

Immediate treatment

Remove and discard tight-fitting shoes. Wear roomier shoes, especially when exercising. Padding the bunion may relieve some of the pain. Anti-inflammatory medication.

Rehabilitation and prevention

Prevention is essential when assessing bunions. Footwear with enough room for the feet will help prevent this condition. Avoiding undue pressure and taking care to treat even minor toe injuries will also prevent bunions. When a bunion does develop, padding the area when exercising will help to alleviate the pain.

Long-term prognosis

Bunions respond to treatment quite well. In cases where the bunion has advanced or it does not respond to treatment, surgery may be needed to correct the condition. Depending on the surgical procedure, recovery may be almost immediate to several weeks.

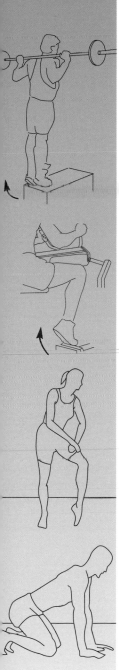

Brief outline of injury

Hammer toe gets its name from the hammer-like or claw-like appearance of the affected toe. The toe bends upward at the first joint and down at the second causing this appearance. Ill-fitting shoes and muscle or nerve damage to the flexor muscle group may result in this condition. Corns and/or calluses may also develop due to the pressure of the toe against the shoes.

Anatomy and physiology

The *proximal phalanx* of a toe (most often that of the second toe) is extended, and the *second* and *distal phalanges* are flexed, forming a hammer-like appearance. This causes pressure on the ball of the foot and causes the mid-toe area to rub against the top of the shoe. This could lead to *corns* or *calluses*. Diabetes, stroke, arthritis, or prior injury could also cause an unnatural flexing of the toes.

Cause of injury

Ill-fitting shoes. Muscle or nerve damage in the flexor muscle group.

Signs and symptoms

Hammer-like appearance of the toe. Pain and difficulty moving the toe. Corns and calluses may develop on the affected toe.

Complications if left unattended

When left unattended, hammer toe can lead to other problems such as arthritis, painful corns and calluses, and flexor tendinitis. It may also lead to a complete inability to extend or straighten the toe.

Immediate treatment

Switch to roomier shoes. Anti-inflammatory medication.

Rehabilitation and prevention

Stretching and strengthening the toes will aid recovery and correct the flexing of the toes if they are still flexible. Selecting properly fitted shoes and stretching the toes regularly will help prevent hammer toe from developing. Straps and padding may be required to relieve some of the pain.

Long-term prognosis

Surgery may be required if the toe has become inflexible and other treatments do not work.

114: TURF TOE

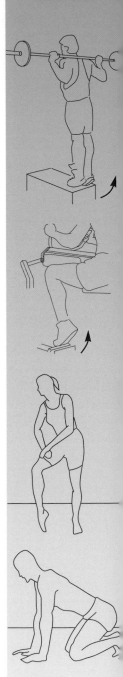

Brief outline of injury

Pain at the base of the big toe may be a result of turf toe. Athletes who jam their toe or repetitively push off when running or jumping are susceptible. Also caused by hyperextending the metatarsophalangeal joint of the great toe. The name turf toe comes from the fact that this injury is common among athletes who play on artificial turf.

Anatomy and physiology

Turf toe develops at the *metatarsophalangeal joint* of the great toe. The capsule that covers this joint is torn, leading to instability and pain. This can lead to dislocations, cartilage wear and eventually arthritis. The tendons that cross the joint can become involved as well. Jamming the toe, or pushing off when running or jumping puts stress on the capsule and can lead to tearing.

Cause of injury

Jamming the toe. Repetitive pushing off on the toe, especially on a harder surface such as artificial turf.

Signs and symptoms

Pain at the base of the toe. Some swelling may be noted in the joint. Pain increases when pushing off with the toe.

Complications if left unattended

Turf toe can lead to chronic pain and the inability to run or jump. When left unattended, turf toe can lead to other conditions such as *toe dislocations* and *arthritis*.

Immediate treatment

Rest. Ice. Anti-inflammatory medication.

Rehabilitation and prevention

As the pain subsides, it is important to work on the strength and flexibility of the toes. Adjusting the way the pressure is applied to the foot when pushing off will also help to correct the condition(s) that caused the turf toe. Alternating workouts from hard to softer surfaces will help prevent the development of this condition. Special inserts, which support the toe may be used when returning to activity. A gradual return to full activity is important.

Long-term prognosis

Turf toe does have a tendency to return when working out on the same surface. In most cases, pain will subside and normal function will return. In very rare cases, surgery is required to alleviate the symptoms.

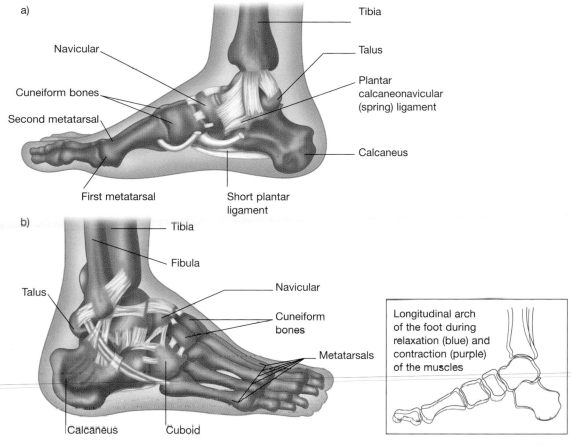

a)

Tibia

Navicular

Talus

Cuneiform bones

Plantar calcaneonavicular (spring) ligament

Second metatarsal

Calcaneus

First metatarsal

Short plantar ligament

b)

Tibia

Fibula

Talus

Navicular

Cuneiform bones

Metatarsals

Calcaneus

Cuboid

Longitudinal arch of the foot during relaxation (blue) and contraction (purple) of the muscles

Figure 17.4: The arches of the right foot; a) medial view, b) lateral view.

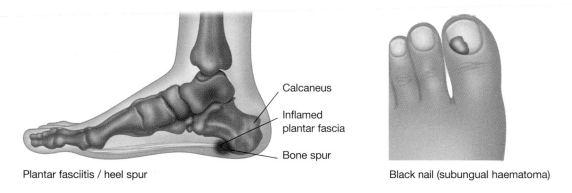

Calcaneus

Inflamed plantar fascia

Bone spur

Plantar fasciitis / heel spur

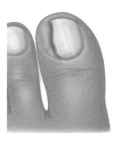

Black nail (subungual haematoma)

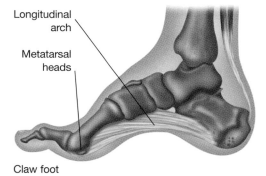

Longitudinal arch

Metatarsal heads

Claw foot

Ingrown toenail

115: CLAW FOOT (PES CAVUS)

Brief outline of injury

Pes cavus (claw foot) is a genetic condition that causes a high arch, giving the foot a claw-like appearance. This often leads to tight calf muscles and pain in the forefoot. People with claw foot have difficulty finding shoes that fit properly, which can lead to other foot conditions. This condition is the opposite of flat feet but is much less common.

Anatomy and physiology

Pes cavus is a condition in which there is exaggerated height of the *longitudinal arch*, which means that the foot is fairly inflexible due to tight calf muscles. This foot positioning puts additional stress on the *metatarsal heads*. The calf tendon is stretched over the heel and into the arch and the raised arch puts additional stress on the calf muscles. Those people with this genetic disorder must work to correct it or work around it in their activities.

Cause of injury

Genetic condition. Possibly secondary to contractures or disturbed balance of the muscles.

Signs and symptoms

Pain in the foot, especially when walking or running. Toes may be bent.

Complications if left unattended

If left unattended, pes cavus can lead to chronic pain and possible injury to other structures in the foot. Foot instability is common, and could lead to strains and sprains.

Immediate treatment

Stretch the calf muscles and the foot. Contact a sports medicine professional if painful and unable to treat.

Rehabilitation and prevention

Stretching the calf muscles and the foot is the first and most important step in rehabilitation. Finding proper fitting shoes will be important as well, which will help support the arch but also prevent injury due to the instability of the foot. Strengthening the muscles of the lower leg will also support the foot. If surgery is required, it will be important to increase strength and flexibility in the muscles that are immobilized.

Long-term prognosis

When treated properly, claw foot can be corrected and the symptoms relieved. Surgery may be an option, especially when pain is severe and other treatments do not help.

Rehabilitation exercises

**Rehabilitation
exercises**

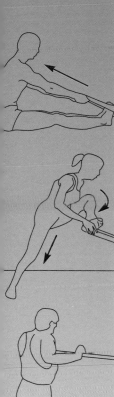

Brief outline of injury

Plantar fasciitis is an injury to the plantar fascia that connects the heel to the base of the toes. Pain is usually felt in the heel especially upon rising from an extended rest. Walking or running, especially on hard surfaces and with tight calf muscles, makes an athlete more susceptible to this injury, as does being female and/or overweight. High or fallen arches and incorrect footwear can lead to this condition as well.

Anatomy and physiology

The plantar fascia, also called *plantar aponeurosis*, is a tough fibrous tissue that originates from the tuberosity of the calcaneus to the metatarsal heads, and is important for supporting the longitudinal arch of the foot. When the calves are tight, this tissue is under stress. Repetitive ankle movement, especially when restricted by tight calves, can irritate this tissue at the calcaneus.

Cause of injury

Tight calf muscles and running on hard surfaces. Improper or ill-fitting footwear. Arch problems. Training errors. Overuse. Hyperpronation. Poor flexibility of the *triceps surae* (*gastrocnemius, soleus,* and *plantaris*) and Achilles tendon.

Signs and symptoms

Pain at the heel bone, which is worse after exercise or when rising from an extended rest. Pain may diminish during exercise, but return after the activity is stopped.

Complications if left unattended

Plantar fasciitis that is left unattended can lead to chronic pain that may cause a change in walking or running gait. This in turn can lead to knee, hip, and lower back problems.

Immediate treatment

Rest. Ice. Ultrasound. Anti-inflammatory medication. Then heat and massage to promote blood flow and healing

Rehabilitation and prevention

Stretching the Achilles tendon and the plantar fascia will help speed recovery and prevent a recurrence. A special orthotic or insert for the shoe may be required at the beginning of the return to activity. Strengthening the muscles of the lower leg will also serve to protect the fascia and prevent this condition.

Long-term prognosis

Most people with plantar fasciitis recover completely after a few weeks to a few months of treatment. Injections of corticosteroid may be necessary in cases where the fascia doesn't respond to early treatment.

SPORTS INJURIES OF THE FOOT

Brief outline of injury

A spur is a hook, or spike of bone, commonly seen on the heel bone (calcaneus). Heel spurs are often associated with plantar fasciitis, although they may be seen without it. Spurs can occur in other bones as well. When a tendon or ligament runs over the spur it causes inflammation and pain. Athletes with previous injuries or irritations of the tendon to bone attachments have a higher risk of bone spurs.

Anatomy and physiology

When a section of bone becomes injured or irritated it will add calcium to the area to strengthen it. These calcium deposits become the *bone spurs*. In the foot, heel spurs can form on the lower surface of the *calcaneus*, and sites where tendons or ligaments attach to bone are more commonly the sites of these spurs. Bone spurs irritate the tendons that cross over them, creating more inflammation within the tendon, which may increase the spur.

Cause of injury

Irritation of the plantar fascia and calcaneal attachment. Untreated minor injury to bones. Calcium deposits on the outside of a healthy bone.

Signs and symptoms

Pain and tenderness at the heel, or other site of the spur. Possible grinding or clicking felt as the tendon crosses the spur.

Complications if left unattended

Bone spurs can cause injury to the tendons that surround them, which causes more inflammation and in turn may worsen the bone spur.

Immediate treatment

Rest from activities that cause pain. Anti-inflammatory medication.

Rehabilitation and prevention

Identifying and correcting the condition that caused the irritation to the plantar fascia or other tendon will help with recovery, and prevent a recurrence. Stretching the muscles and tendons involved will also speed recovery. The use of a *heel cup, heel cradle* or other orthotic device to reduce the stress on the plantar fascia may also help when returning to activity. Making sure to treat even minor injuries will also help prevent bone spurs.

Long-term prognosis

Heel spurs should respond well to rest and rehabilitation. Some may require orthotics to alleviate the symptoms and aid recovery. If the bone spur doesn't respond to treatment, it would have to be surgically removed to prevent future damage.

Rehabilitation exercises

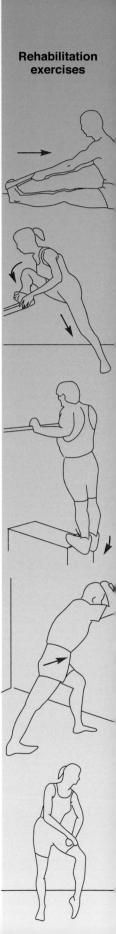

Brief outline of injury

A subungual haematoma is bleeding under the toenail caused by an injury or infection to the nail bed. Crushing injury is the most common mechanism for this type of injury. The bleeding under the nail causes pressure and pain to the nail bed. The pocket of blood may be small or cover the whole area under the nail.

Anatomy and physiology

The nail protects the area under the toenail, the *nail bed*, but when crushing trauma, an object under the nail, or infection causes damage to this soft area, bleeding may occur. Because the nail is a hard surface, it holds the blood in and this bleeding causes pressure and pain. Depending on the initial injury, the bone underneath may also be involved.

Cause of injury

Crushing injury to the toe. Foreign object under the nail causing a laceration to the nail bed. Infection under the nail causing bleeding.

Signs and symptoms

Pain and pressure under the nail. Red, maroon or other dark colour under the nail.

Complications if left unattended

The bleeding and resulting pressure under the nail may cause damage to the underlying tissues, killing them over time. The nail may fall off and this could lead to infection if not treated properly. If the bone was fractured during the initial injury, chronic pain may result.

Immediate treatment

Rest, ice, and elevation. If the nail comes off, it is important to keep it covered and protected. If the possibility of a fracture exists, such as with a crushing injury, seek medical attention.

Rehabilitation and prevention

The nail may need to be removed during treatment, or may fall off on its own, leaving the nail bed exposed. It is important to keep this area protected to prevent infection. It is also important to protect the affected toe while it is healing. Padding over the toes may be needed. Avoiding impact to the toes and protecting them during activities will help prevent this injury.

Long-term prognosis

A subungual haematoma will usually respond well to treatment, although in cases involving more than 25% of the nail bed and pressure that is unrelieved by initial treatments, a physician may need to drain the blood from the nail bed. If an infection is the cause, oral or topical antibiotics may be required.

Brief outline of injury

Ingrown (ingrowing) toenails can be very painful. They are the result of trauma to the toe, tight-fitting shoes, or improper grooming of the toenails. Pain and infection may result from the skin growing over the nail or the nail growing into the skin on the sides. Redness and swelling on the outside of the toe may also be noted.

Anatomy and physiology

The toenail is a horny cutaneous plate, which normally grows outward away from the base of the toe. It is made up of epithelial scales developed from the *stratum lucidum* of the skin. If the nail is cut or broken too low, it may grow into the skin on the side of the toe, or the skin may grow over the toenail. Injury to the toe, such as stubbing the toe or even a toe fracture, can cause the toenail to grow into the skin. Tight-fitting shoes may also put pressure on the outside of the toe pressing skin into the nail and causing it to grow over the nail. When the skin grows into or over the nail, an environment develops that is ripe for infection.

Cause of injury

Trauma to the toe, such as stubbing the toe. Tight or improperly fitting shoes. Improper toenail grooming techniques.

Signs and symptoms

Pain. Redness and swelling in the affected area. Pus or other signs of infection may be present.

Complications if left unattended

If left unattended, an ingrown toenail may become infected and the infection may eventually involve the entire toe, or even the foot. The pain may become chronic and affect the ability to wear certain shoes. Athlete may develop a limp.

Immediate treatment

Soak the foot in warm water. Get rid of the tight-fitting shoes and select roomier ones. Keep the feet dry during the day. Seek the assistance of a qualified podiatrist.

Rehabilitation and prevention

When treating the ingrown nail, it is important to protect it from additional trauma or injury. Change socks as needed to keep the feet dry. Wearing shoes with plenty of room for the toes will aid healing and prevent further ingrown toenails. Protecting the toes from trauma will also help prevent this condition. After trauma to the toe it is important to check the toenails for breakage and pressing of the nail into the skin.

Long-term prognosis

Ingrown toenails commonly respond to treatment and repair completely. Ingrown toenails may become a recurring problem in some cases, especially if the underlying causes are not addressed. In cases where infection has set in and does not respond to initial treatment, surgery may be required. Removal of all or part of the toenail and the infected tissue may be required.

Glossary of Terms

Abrasion Skin wound in which the external layers have been rubbed/scraped off.

Achilles tendinitis Inflammation of the Achilles tendon.

Acute injury Injury from a specific event, leading to a sudden onset of symptoms.

Adhesive capsulitis Adhesive inflammation between the joint capsule and the peripheral articular cartilage of the shoulder. Causes pain, stiffness, and limitation of movement. Also known as frozen shoulder syndrome.

Angina Any spasmodic, choking, or suffocative pain, e.g. preceding a myocardial infarction (heart attack).

Ankylosing spondylitis Form of degenerative joint disease that affects the spine. Systemic illness, producing pain and stiffness as a result of inflammation of the sacroiliac, intervertebral, and costovertebral joints.

Anterior tibial compartment syndrome Rapid swelling, increased tension, and pain of the anterior tibial compartment of the leg. Usually a history of eixcessive exertion.

Aortic aneurysm Sac formed by the dilation of the wall of the aorta, which is filled with fluid or clotted blood.

Apley's scratch test Determines range of motion: internal rotation and adduction; internal rotation, extension, and adduction; abduction, flexion, and external rotation.

Arteritis Inflammation of an artery.

Arthropathy Any joint disease.

Atrophy A wasting away or deterioration of tissue due to disease, disuse, or malnutrition.

Articular dysfunction Disturbance, impairment, or abnormality of a joint.

Avulsion fracture Indirect fracture caused by compressive forces from direct trauma or excessive tensile forces.

Baker's cyst Swelling behind the knee, caused by leakage of synovial fluid which has become enclosed in a sac of membrane.

Blister Fluid accumulation under the skin caused by friction of the skin over a hard or rough surface, causing the epidermis to separate from the dermis.

Bunion Abnormal prominence of the inner aspect of the first metatarsal head, resulting in displacement of the great toe (hallux valgus).

Bursa Fibrous sac membrane containing synovial fluid, typically found between tendons and bones. It acts to reduce friction during movement.

Bursitis Inflammation of the bursa, e.g. subdeltoid bursa.

Calcific tendinitis Inflammation and calcification of the subacromial or subdeltoid bursa. This results in pain, and limitation of movement of the shoulder.

Callus Localized thickening of skin epidermis due to physical trauma.

Cancellous Bone tissue of relatively low density.

Capsulitis Inflammation of a capsule, e.g. joint.

Cardiac arrhythmia Variation from the normal rhythm of the heartbeat.

Carpal tunnel syndrome Compression of the median nerve as it passes through the carpal tunnel, leading to pain and tingling in the hand.

Cauliflower ear Haematoma between the perichondrium and cartilage of the outer ear.

Chondral fracture Fracture involving the articular cartilage at a joint.

Chondromalacia patellae Degenerative condition in the articular cartilage of the patella caused by abnormal compression or shearing forces.

Chronic injury Injury characterized by a slow, sustained development of symptoms that culminates in a painful inflammatory condition.

Claw toe Toe deformity, particularly in patients with rheumatoid arthritis, consisting of dorsal subluxation of toes 2–5; painful condition during walking. The patient develops a shuffling gait.

Coccydynia Pain in the coccyx and neighbouring region. Also known as coccygodynia.

Collateral ligaments Major ligaments that cross the medial and lateral aspects of the knee.

Colles' fracture Fracture of the radius and ulna, just proximal to the wrist, that results in the distal segment displacing in a dorsal and radial direction.

Compressive force Axial loading that produces a squeezing effect on a structure.

Compartment syndrome Condition in which increased intramuscular pressure impedes blood flow and function of tissues within that compartment.

Concussion Violent shaking or jarring action of the brain, resulting in immediate or transient impairment of neurological function.

Contracture Adhesions occurring in an immobilized muscle, leading to a shortened contractile state.

Contraindication A condition adversely affected by a specific action.

Contusion Compression injury involving accumulation of blood and lymph within a muscle. Also known as a bruise.

Cruciate ligaments Major ligaments that criss-cross the knee in the anteroposterior direction.

Deep vein thrombosis (DVT) The formation of a stationary blood clot in the wall of one or more of the deep veins of the lower leg.

De Quervain's tenosynovitis Inflammatory narrowing tenosynovitis of the abductor pollicis longus and extensor pollicis brevis tendons.

Diffuse injury Injury over a large body area, usually due to low-velocity–high-mass forces.

Discogenic pain Pain caused by derangement of an intervertebral disc.

Discopathy Disease of an intervertebral cartilage (disc).

Dupuytren's contracture Shortening, thickening, and fibrosis of the palmar fascia, producing a flexion deformity of a finger/toe.

Dysmenorrhoea Difficult or painful menstruation.

Dyspnoea Breathlessness or shortness of breath.

Efferent nerves Nerves carrying stimuli from the central nervous system to the muscles.

Epicondylitis Inflammation and microrupturing of the soft tissues on the epicondyles of the distal humerus.

Epiphyseal fracture Injury to the growth plate of a long bone in children and adolescents; may lead to arrested bone growth.

Erythema Redness of the skin produced by congestion of the capillaries.

Fasciitis Inflammation of the fascia surrounding portions of a muscle.

Fibromyalgia Pain and stiffness in the muscles and joints that is either diffuse or has multiple trigger points.

Fracture A disruption in the continuity of a bone.

Frozen shoulder syndrome See adhesive capsulitis.

Ganglion cyst Benign tumour mass commonly seen on the dorsal aspect of the wrist.

Golfer's elbow Inflammation of the medial epicondyle of the humerus caused by activities (e.g. golf) that involve gripping and twisting, especially when there is a forceful grip.

Haematoma Localized mass of blood and lymph confined within a space or tissue.

Hallux The first, or great, toe.

Hallux rigidus Painful flexion deformity of the great toe, in which there is limitation of motion at the metatarsophalangeal joint.

Hallux valgus Angulation of the great toe away from the midline of the body, or toward the other toes.

Hammer toe Flexion deformity of the distal interphalangeal (DIP) joint of the toes.

Heel spur Bony spur from the calcaneum.

Hemiplegia Paralysis of one side of the body.

Hernia Protrusion of abdominal viscera through a weakened portion of the abdominal wall.

Hip pointer Contusions caused by direct compression to an unprotected iliac crest that crushes soft tissue and, sometimes, the bone itself.

Iliotibial band syndrome Pain / inflammation of the iliotibial band, a non-elastic collagen cord stretching from the pelvis to below the knee. There are various biomechanical causes.

Impingement syndrome Chronic condition caused by a repetitive overhead activity that damages the glenoid labrum, long head of the biceps brachii, and subacromial bursa.

Inflammation Pain, swelling, redness, heat, and loss of function that accompany musculo-skeletal injuries.

Innvervation Nerve supply to a body part.

Ischemia Local anaemia due to decreased blood supply.

Laceration Wound that may leave a smooth or jagged edge through the skin, subcutaneous tissues, muscles, and associated nerves and blood vessels.

Larson-Johansson syndrome Inflammation or partial avulsion of the apex of the patella due to traction forces.

Lesion Any pathological or traumatic discontinuity of tissue or loss of function of a part.

Lordosis Excessive convex curve in the lumbar region of the spine.

Mallet finger Rupture of the extensor tendon from the distal phalanx, due to forceful flexion of the phalanx.

McBurney's point Site one-third the distance between the anterior superior iliac spine (ASIS) and umbilicus that, with deep palpation, produces rebound tenderness, indicating appendicitis.

Menisci Fibrocartilagenous discs within the knee that reduce joint stress.

Meralgia paresthetica Entrapment of the lateral femoral cutaneous nerve at the inguinal ligament, causing pain and numbness of the outer surface of the thigh in the region supplied by the nerve.

Metatarsalgia Condition involving general discomfort around the metatarsal's heads.

Microtrauma Injury to a small number of cells due to accumulative effects of repetitive forces.

Morton's neuralgia Form of foot pain, metatarsalgia caused by compression of a branch of the plantar nerve by the metatarsal heads.

Morton's neuroma Tumour growing from a nerve or made up largely of nerve cells and nerve fibres, resulting from Morton's neuralgia.

Muscle spindle Encapsulated receptor found in muscle tissue sensitive to stretch.

Myositis Inflammation of connective tissues within a muscle.

Myositis ossificans Accumulation of mineral deposits in muscle tissue.

Neuritis Inflammation of a nerve, with pain and tenderness.

Neurogenic Forming nervous tissue, or originating in the nervous system.

Neuropathy Functional disturbance or pathological change in the peripheral nervous system.

Nonunion fracture A fracture in which healing is delayed or fails to unite at all.

NSAID Nonsteroidal anti-inflammatory drug.

Oedema Accumulation of lymphatic fluid in the tissues, caused by failure of the lymphatic system to drain properly.

Osgood-schlatter syndrome Inflammation or partial avulsion of the tibial apophysis due to traction forces.

Osteitis Inflammation of a bone, causing enlargement of the bone, tenderness, and a dull, aching pain.

Osteoarthritis Noninflammatory degenerative joint disease, characterized by degeneration of the articular cartilage, hypertrophy of bone at the margins, and changes in the synovial membrane. Seen particularly in older persons.

Osteochondritis dissecans Localized area of avascular necrosis resulting from complete or incomplete separation of joint cartilage and subchondral bone.

Overuse injury Any injury caused by excessive, repetitive movement of the body part.

Paget's disease Rare disease where bone is replaced by fibrous tissue that then becomes hard and brittle, with much pain. Particularly affecting the skull, spine, and leg bones.

Painful arc syndrome Pain located within a limited number of degrees in the range of motion.

Paralysis Partial or complete loss of the ability to move a body part.

Passive stretching Stretching of muscles, tendons, and ligaments produced by a stretching force other than tension in the anagonist muscles.

Patellofemoral stress syndrome Condition whereby the lateral retinaculum is tight or the vastus medialis oblique is weak, leading to lateral excursion and pressure on the lateral facet of the patella, causing a painful condition.

Pes cavus High arch.

Pes planus Flat feet.

Plantar fascia Specialized band of fascia that covers the plantar surface of the foot and helps support the longitudinal arch.

Plyometric training Exercises that employ explosive movements to develop muscular power.

Posterior compartment syndrome Pain in the posterior compartment of the lower leg, including soleus, gastrocnemius, tibialis posterior, flexor digitorum longus, and flexor hallucis longus. Site of pain varies depending on muscles affected.

Prognosis Probable cause or progress of injury.

Propriceptors Specialized deep sensory nerve cells in joints, ligaments, muscles, and tendons sensitive to stretch, tension, and pressure, which are responsible for position and movement.

Q-angle Angle between the line of quadriceps force and the patellar (tendon) ligament.

Radiculopathy Disease of the nerve roots.

Referred pain Pain felt in a region of the body other than where the source or actual cause of the pain is located.

Repetitive strain injury (RSI) Refers to any overuse condition, such as strain, or tendonitis in any part of the body.

Rheumatoid arthritis Autoimmune disease, in which the immune system attacks the body's own tissues. Causes inflammation of many parts of the body.

Rotator cuff The SITS (supraspinatus, infraspinatus, teres minor, and subscapularis) muscles that hold the head of the humerus in the glenoid fossa and produce humeral rotation.

Sacroiliitis Inflammation (arthritis) in the sacroiliac joint.

Scapulocostal syndrome Pain in the superior or posterior aspect of the shoulder girdle, as a result of long-standing alteration of the relationship of the scapula and the posterior thoracic wall.

Sciatica Compression of a spinal nerve due to a herniated disc, a muscle-related or facet joint disease, or compression between the two parts of the piriformis.

Scoliosis Lateral rotational spinal curvature.

Seronegative spondyloarthropathy A general term comprising a number of degenerative joint diseases having common features, e.g. synovitis of the peripheral joints.

Sesamoid bones Short bones embedded in tendons; largest is the patella.

Sesamoiditis Inflammation of the sesamoid bones of the first metatarsal.

Sever's disease A traction-type injury, or osteochondrosis, of the calcaneal apophysis, seen in young adolescents.

Shear force A force that acts parallel or tangent to a plane passing through an object.

Snapping hip syndrome A snapping sensation either heard or felt during motion at the hip.

Somatic pain Pain originating in the skin, ligaments, muscles, bones, or joints.

Spasm Transitory muscle contractions.

Spondyloarthropathy Disease of the joints of the spine.

Spondylolisthesis Forward displacement of one vertebra over another.

Spondylolysis Dissolution of a vertebra.

Spondylosis Degenerative spinal changes due to osteoarthritis.

Sprain Injury to ligamentous tissue.

Static stretch Slow, sustained muscle stretching used to increase flexibility.

Stenosis Abnormal narrowing of a duct or canal, e.g. spinal stenosis, a narrowing of the vertebral canal, caused by encroachment of the bone upon the space.

Strain Amount of deformation with respect to the original dimensions of the structure.

Stress The distribution of force within a body.

Stress (march) fracture Hairline crack of a bone caused by excessive repetitive stress.

Subungual haematoma Collection of blood under the nail, caused by direct trauma.

Synovitis Inflammation of a synovial membrane, particularly a joint.

Tendinopathy Disease of a tendon.
Tendinitis Inflammation of a tendon. Also known as tendonitis.
Tennis elbow Tendonitis of the muscles of the back of the forearm at their insertion and is caused by excessive hammering or sawing type movements, or a tense, awkward grip on a tennis racquet.
Tenosynovitis Inflammation of a tendon sheath.
Thoracic outlet syndrome Compression of the brachial plexus rather than the nerve roots, and so symptoms appear in the arm instead of the neck.
Thrombophlebitis Inflammation of a vein, associated with thrombus formation.
Thrombus Stationary blood clot along the wall of a blood vessel, frequently causing vascular obstruction.

Volkmann's contracture Ischemic necrosis of the forearm muscles and tissues, caused by damage to the blood flow.

Anatomical Directions

Abduction A movement away from the midline (or to return from adduction).
Adduction A movement toward the midline (or to return from abduction).
Anatomical position The body is upright with the arms and hands turned forward.
Anterior Towards the front of the body (as opposed to posterior).

Circumduction Movement in which the distal end of a bone moves in a circle, while the proximal end remains stable.
Contralateral On the opposite side.
Coronal plane A vertical plane at right angles to the sagittal plane that divides the body into anterior and posterior portions.

Deep Away from the surface (as opposed to superficial).
Depression Movement of an elevated part of the body downwards to its original position.
Distal Away from the point of origin of a structure (as opposed to proximal).
Dorsal Relating to the back or posterior portion (as opposed to ventral).

Elevation Movement of a part of the body upwards along the frontal plane.
Eversion To turn the sole of the foot outward.
Extension A movement at a joint resulting in separation of two ventral surfaces (as opposed to flexion).

Flexion A movement at a joint resulting in approximation of two ventral surfaces (as opposed to extension).

Horizontal plane A transverse plane at right angle to the long axis of the body.

Inferior Below or furthest away from the head.
Inversion To turn the sole of the foot inward.

Lateral Located away from the midline (opposite to medial).

Medial Situated close to or at the midline of the body or organ (opposite to lateral).
Median Centrally located, situated in the middle of the body.

Opposition A movement specific to the saddle joint of the thumb, that enables you to touch your thumb to the tips of the fingers of the same hand.

Palmar Anterior surface of the hand.
Plantar The sole of the foot.
Posterior Relating to the back or the dorsal aspect of the body (opposite to anterior).
Pronation To turn the palm of the hand down to face the floor, or away from the anatomical and foetal positions.
Prone Position of the body in which the ventral surface faces down (as opposed to supine).
Protraction Movement forwards in the transverse plane.
Proximal Closer to the centre of the body or to the point of attachment of a limb.

Retraction Movement backwards in the transverse plane.
Rotation Move around a fixed axis.

Sagittal plane A vertical plane extending in an antero-posterior direction dividing the body into right and left parts.
Superficial On or near the surface (as opposed to deep).
Superior Above or closest to the head.
Supination To turn the palm of the hand up to face the ceiling, or toward the anatomical and foetal positions.
Supine Position of the body in which the ventral surface faces up (as opposed to prone).

Ventral Refers to the anterior part of the body (as opposed to dorsal).

The Seven Types of Synovial Joints

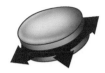

Plane or Gliding
Movement occurs when two, generally flat or slightly curved surfaces glide across one another. Examples: the acromioclavicular joint, and the sacroiliac joint.

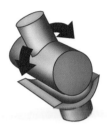

Hinge
Movement occurs around only one axis; a transverse one, as in the hinge of the lid of a box. A protrusion of one bone fits into a concave or cylindrical articular surface of another, permitting flexion and extension. Examples: the interphalangeal joints, the elbow, and the knee.

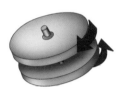

Pivot
Movement takes place around a vertical axis, like the hinge of a gate. A more or less cylindrical articular surface of bone protrudes into and rotates within a ring formed by bone or ligament. Example: the joint between the radius and the ulna at the elbow.

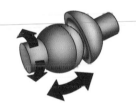

Ball-and-socket
Consists of a 'ball' formed by the spherical or hemispherical head of one bone that rotates within the concave 'socket' of another, allowing flexion, extension, adduction, abduction, circumduction, and rotation. Thus, they are multiaxial and allow the greatest range of movement of all joints. Examples: the shoulder and the hip joints.

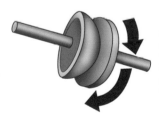

Condyloid
Have a spherical articular surface that fits into a matching concavity. Permits flexion, extension, abduction, adduction, and circumduction. Example: the metacarpophalangeal joints of the fingers (but not the thumb).

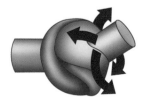

Saddle
Articulating surfaces have convex and concave areas, and so resemble two 'saddles' that join them together by accommodating each other's convex to concave surfaces. Allow even more movement than condyloid joints, for example, allowing the 'opposition' of the thumb to the fingers. Example: the carpometacarpal joint of the thumb.

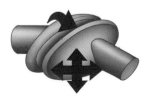

Ellipsoid
An ellipsoid joint is effectively similar to a ball-and-socket joint, but the articular surfaces are ellipsoid instead of spherical, allowing flexion, extension, adduction, abduction, and circumduction. Example: the radiocarpal joint.

Resources

Anderson, D.M. (chief lexicographer): 2003. *Dorland's Illustrated Medical Dictionary, 30th edition.* Saunders, an imprint of Elsevier, Philadelphia, USA

Anderson, M.K. & Hall, S.J.: 1997. *Fundamentals of Sports Injury Management.* Williams & Wilkins, Baltimore, USA

Arnheim, D.D.: 1989. *Modern Principles of Athletic Training.* Times Mirror, MO, USA

Bahr, R. & Maehlum, S.: 2004. *Clinical Guide to Sports Injuries.* Human Kinetics, IL, USA

Delavier, F.: 2001. *Strength Training Anatomy.* Human Kinetics, IL, USA

Dornan, P. & Dunn, R.: 1988. *Sporting Injuries.* University of Queensland Press, Qld, Australia

Jarmey, C.: 2003. *The Concise Book of Muscles.* Lotus Publishing. Chichester, UK/ North Atlantic Books, Berkeley, USA

Jarmey, C.: 2006. *The Concise Book of the Moving Body.* Lotus Publishing, Chichester, UK/ North Atlantic Books, Berkeley, USA

Klossner, D.: 2006. *NCAA Sports Medicine Handbook.* The National Collegiate Athletic Association, IN, USA

Lamb, D.R.: 1984. *Physiology of Exercise.* Macmillan Publishing Co., NY, USA

Levy, A.M. & Fuerst, M.L.: 1993. *Sports Injury Handbook.* John Wiley & Sons, Inc., NY, USA

Micheli, L.J.: 1995. *Sports Medicine Bible.* HarperCollins Publishers, Inc., NY, USA

Norris, C.M.: 1998. *Sports Injuries: Diagnosis and Management.* Butterworth Heinemann, Oxford, UK

Reid, M.G.: 1994. *Sports Medicine Awareness Course.* Sports Medicine Australia, ACT, Australia

Rushall, B.S. & Pyke, F.S.: 1990. *Training for Sports and Fitness.* Macmillan Education Australia, NSW, Australia

S.M.A.: 1986. *The Sports Trainer.* Jacaranda Press, Qld, Australia

Tortora, G.J. & Anagnostakos, N.P.: 1990. *Principles of Anatomy and Physiology.* Harper & Row, NY, USA

Walker, B.E.: 1998. *The Stretching Handbook.* Walkerbout Health, Qld, Australia

Walker, B.E.: 2006. *The Sports Injury Handbook.* Walkerbout Health, Qld, Australia

Walker, B.E.: 2007. *The Anatomy of Stretching.* Lotus Publishing, Chichester, UK/ North Atlantic Books, Berkeley, USA

Index

Abrasions 55
Accidents 51
Acetabulum 165, 175
Achilles tendon 205–207, 228, 241
Acromioclavicular joint 121, 122
Acromion 117, 122, 131
Acute cervical disc disease, see slipped disc
Acute torticollis, see wryneck
Adhesive capsulitis, see frozen shoulder
Aloe vera 56
Anabolic steroids 109
Anconeus 110
Annular ligament 105, 106
Annulus pulposus 73, 143, 144
Anterior compartment syndrome 211
Anterior intercondylar area 188
Anterior talofibular ligament 215
Aponeurosis 100
Apophyses 159
Arthritis 238
Articular (hyaline) cartilage 199
Athlete's foot 59
Auditory canal 79
Auditory ossicles 79
Avascular necrosis 195
Avulsion 109

Balance, see proprioception
Bankart lesion 119
Biceps brachii 125–127
Biceps femoris 178, 179
Biomechanical error 51
Black nail 118
Blisters 60
Blood pooling 17
Bone 9
Bone spurs 75, 130, 242
Brachial plexus 68
Bruise 65, 67, 126, 141, 179
Bulging disc 144
Bunionette 236
Bunions 236
Burner syndrome, see cervical nerve
  stretch syndrome
Bursa(e) 11
Bursectomy 114
Bursitis 114, 131, 171, 181, 191, 228

Calcaneofibular ligament 215
Calcaneus 222, 224, 227–229, 242
Calluses 61, 237
Cancellous bone 203
Capitate 83
Capitulum 105
Carpal bones 94
Carpal tunnel syndrome 97
Carpometacarpal joint 87, 88
Cartilage 10
Cartilaginous septum 80
Cauliflower ear 79
Cementum 77
Cervical nerve stretch syndrome 68
Cervical radiculitis, see pinched nerve
Cervical spine 67
Cervical spondylosis, see bone spurs
Chafing 55
Chondromalacia patellae 196, 199
Circuit training 26
Clavicle 117, 127
Claw foot 240
Collar bone, see clavicle
Colles' fracture 93
Concentric muscle contraction 31
Concussion 65
Conditioning 51
Condyles 203, 210
Contusion, see bruise
Cool-down 17
Coracoclavicular joint 121
Cornea 78
Corns 61, 237
Cross training 28
Cuts 55

Deep infrapatellar bursa 191
Delayed-onset muscle soreness (DOMS) 17
Deltoid 122
Deltoid ligament 215
Dentin 77
De Quervain's tendovaginitis 101
Dermatophytes 59
Dermis 55
Diabetes mellitus 89, 109
Dislocation 88, 95, 107, 119, 238
Dorsal ligaments 95
Dura mater 65

Ear   79
Eccentric muscle contraction   30
Ecchymosis   141
Enamel   77
Entrapment neuropathies   97
Epidermis   55
Epistaxis   80
Ethmoid   80
Eustachian tube   79
Extensor digitorum longus   231
Extensor hallucis longus   231
Extensors   139
Eye   78

Facilities   42
Fascia   211
Femoral condyles   196, 200
Femur   175
Fibrinoid necrosis   89
Fibula   203, 216, 222, 224, 227
Fitness   22
FITT principle   19
Flail chest   151
Flexibility   33
Flexor hallucis brevis   231
Flexor hallucis longus   231
Flexors   139
Fracture   65,67, 83, 93,105,117,145,149
                    163,175, 203, 210, 216, 227, 229
Free weights   24
Frostbite   57
Frozen shoulder   135

Gerdy's tubercle   181
Glenohumeral joint   121,130
Glenoid fossa   117
Glenoid labrum   135
Golfer's elbow   111
Growth plate   159

Haematoma   65
Haemorrhage   65
Hallux valgus   236
Hamate   83
Hammer toe   237
Hamstrings   178,179
Heel spur   242
Herniated disc, see slipped disc
Hills-Sachs lesion   119
Hip pointer   158
Humerus   107,113,117,131

Iliac crest   158
Iliopsoas   157,167
Iliotibial band   169,181
Impingement syndrome   129
Inferior glenohumeral ligament   119
Ingrown toenail   244
Injuries   11
Intercarpal joint   95
Intermetacarpal joint   87
Interphalangeal joint   87, 88
Isometric muscle contraction   31

Joints   10
Jumper's knee, see patellar tendinitis

Knee synovial plica   192

Lacunae   9
Lamellae   109
Larsen-johansson syndrome   193
Lateral epicondyle   110
Lateral femoral condyle   188
Lateral malleolus   215, 219, 220
Ligaments   11
Ligamentum flava   140
Ligamentum nuchae   140
Linea aspera   181
Long extensor tendon   85
Longitudinal arch   240
Lunate   93, 95

Machine weights   23
Mallet finger   85
Medial condyle   187
Medial epicondyle   98,187
Medial epicondylitis, see golfer's elbow
Medial malleolus   215–217
Medial meniscus   187
Medial tibial pain syndrome   209
Median nerve   97, 98
Melanocytes   56
Melanoma   56
Meniscus   189
Metacarpophalangeal joint   87, 88, 236, 238
Metatarsals   227, 229, 233, 240
Morton's neuroma   233
Muscles   8
Myositis ossificans   179
Myxomatous degeneration   89

Nail bed   243
Nasal septum   80

Navicular	93,217	Radial collateral ligament	106,107
Nose	80	Radial nerves	98
Nucleation	61	Radio-carpal joint	95
Nucleus pulposus	73,143,144	Radio-ulnar joint	105
		Radius	105,107,113
Obliques	139,154	Range of motion	48
Olecranon	98,114	Rectus abdominis	154
Olecranon bursa	114	Rectus femoris	157,177,179
Osgood-schlatter syndrome	193	Rehabilitation	46
Osteitis pubis	162	Remodeling	145
Osteochondritis dissecans	195, 222	Retrocalcaneal bursa	206, 228
Osteophytes, see bone formation		Rheumatoid arthritis	89
Overload	51	Ribs	149
Overtraining	20	Rider's strain	160
Own body weight exercises	24	Rotator cuff	129
		Rotators	139
Paratenons	133	Rules	42
Pars interarticularis	145	Runner's knee, see chondromalacia patellae	
Patellar ligament	5,183,197	Ruptured disc, see slipped disc	
Patellar tendon, see patellar ligament			
Patellofemoral groove	196, 200	Scaphoid	93, 95
Patellofemoral joint	196, 200	Scapulothoracic joint	121
Patellofemoral pain syndrome	196	Semimembranosus	178,179
Pectoralis major	127,134	Semitendinosus	178,179
Pelvis	159	Separation	122,123
Peroneus brevis	219, 220	Sesamoiditis	234
Peroneus longus	219, 220	Shin splints, see medial tibial pain syndrome	
Pes anserinus bursa	191	Shoulder girdle	121
Pes cavus, see claw foot		Shoulder joint	121
Phalanges	227, 237	Six-pack	154
Pinched nerve	74	Skeleton	9
Pinna	79	Skier's thumb	84
Piriformis syndrome	165	Skill development	22
Plantar aponeurosis	241	Slipped disc	143
Plantar fascia, see plantar aponeurosis		Snapping hip syndrome	169
Plantar fasciitis	241	Soft pulp	77
Plantar nerve	233	Spinal canal	143,144
Plantar warts	61	Spondylolisthesis	145
Playing areas	42	Spondylolysis	145
Plica	192	Sports injury management	44
Plyometric training	30	Sprain	12,69, 84, 87, 94,106,140, 215
Popliteal fossa	205	Sternoclavicular joint	121,123
Posture	41	Strain	12,139,177,178, 206
Prolotherapy	119	Stratum lucidum	244
Pronation	126, 224	Strength training	23,48
Proprioception	49	Stretching	15,33,48
Protective devices	42	Subacromial bursa	129–131
Pubic symphysis	162	Subcutaneous calcaneal bursa	206
		Subcutaneous prepatellar bursa	191
Q-angle	196	Subluxation	107,121, 200, 219
Quadrangular cartilage	80	Subperichondrial space	80
Quadriceps	177,179	Subtalar joint	223, 224

Subungual haematoma, see black nail

Sunburn 56

Superficial infrapatellar bursa 191

Supination 126, 223

Supinator 110

Suprapatellar bursa 191

Synovial cyst, see wrist ganglion cyst

Synovial fluid 10,135

Synovial hernia, see wrist ganglion cyst

Synovial joints 251

Synovial membrane 192

Talus 216, 222

Teeth 77

Tendinitis 89,101,130,167,168,183 197, 207, 217, 220, 231

Tendons 11,100

Tennis elbow 110

Tenosynovitis 101

Tenosynovium 101

Thera-band 23

Thrower's elbow 113

Tibia 203, 216, 222, 224, 227

Tibialis anterior 211

Tibial tuberosity 193,197, 203, 210

Tinea pedis, see athlete's foot

Transcutaneous electrical nerve stimulation (TENS) 47

Transversus abdominis 154

Trapezium 83

Trapezoid 83

Triceps brachii tendon 109

Triceps surae 205, 241

Triquestral 93, 95

Trochanteric bursa 171

Trochlea 105

Turf toe 238

Tympanic membrane 79

Ulna 105,107,113

Ulnar collateral ligament 84,106,107

Ulnar tunnel syndrome 98

Ultrasound 47

Vastus intermedius 177,179

Vastus lateralis 177,179, 200

Vastus medialis 177,179, 200

Verrucae 61

Vertebrae 143,144

Volar plate 87

Vomer 80

Warm-up 14

Whiplash 69

Wrist ganglion cyst 100

Wryneck 71